A route out of poverty?

Disabled people, work and welfare reform

Edited by Gabrielle Preston

CPAG
94 White Lion Street
London N1 9PF

CPAG promotes action for the relief, directly or indirectly, of poverty among children and families with children. We work to ensure that those on low incomes get their full entitlements to welfare benefits. In our campaigning and information work we seek to improve benefits and policies for low-income families in order to eradicate the injustice of poverty. If you are not already supporting us, please consider making a donation, or ask for details of our membership schemes and publications.

Poverty Publication 114

Published by CPAG
94 White Lion Street, London N1 9PF

Registered Company No. 1993854
Charity No. 294841

A CIP record for this book is available from the British Library

ISBN10: 1 901698 93 9
ISBN13: 978 1 901698 93 0

Cover and design by Devious Designs 0114 2755634
Typeset by Boldface 020 7253 2014
Printed by Russell Press 0115 9784505
Cover photos by Louis Quail/Photofusion, Ulrike Preuss/Photofusion, Paul Doyle/Photofusion

For Mathew

Acknowledgements

I am very grateful to all the people who contributed to this book. Particular thanks are due to Roy Sainsbury, Adrian Sinfield and Paul Dornan for their helpful comments. I am indebted to Michele Wates, who provided detailed comments on the draft, and circulated information to those individuals and organisations who are part of the Social Care Institute for Excellence Supporting Disabled Parents Knowledge Review, who kindly put me in touch with disabled parents who were willing to be interviewed. I would like to thank John Keep and the Disabled Parent Network for their help and support. I am particularly grateful to the families I interviewed for being so generous with their time and for discussing their experiences so openly. Finally, thanks to Alison Key for editing and managing the production of this report.

Gabrielle Preston

About the authors

Tania Burchardt is Academic Fellow at the Centre for Analysis of Social Exclusion at the London School of Economics.

Richard Olsen was Research Fellow in the Nuffield Community Care Studies Unit at the University of Leicester and is now a mental health adviser.

Guy Palmer is Director of the New Policy Institute and co-author of *Monitoring Poverty and Social Exclusion*.

Gabrielle Preston is Policy and Research Officer at CPAG.

Hugh Stickland is an employment adviser in the Economic and Labour Market Division at the Department for Work and Pensions.

Contents

Definition of disability

Although there are problems in the definition of disability, most government statistics use the definition of disability in the Disability Discrimination Act 1995:

> A person has a disability for the purposes of this Act if he has a physical or mental impairment which has a substantial and long-term adverse effect on his ability to carry out normal day-to-day activities.

More recently, the Government in *Improving the Life Chances of Disabled People* widens the definition to:

> Disadvantage experienced by an individual...resulting from barriers to independent living or educational, employment or other opportunities...that impact on people with impairments and/or ill health. A clear distinction needs to be made between disability, impairment and ill-health. Impairments are long-term characteristics of an individual that affect their functioning and/or appearance. Ill-health is the short-term or long-term consequence of disease or sickness.

Foreword

Putting disability at the heart of public policy

In January 2006, the Disability Rights Commission published *Changing Britain for Good: putting disability at the heart of public policy*. We pointed out that across a whole raft of core government targets, including full employment, skills, and building strong, safe and sustainable communities, failure to account properly for the experience of disabled people is increasingly likely to mean failure to deliver in the round. No more can this be said than in relation to child poverty.

A quarter of all children living in income poverty have a disabled parent, and in almost 70 per cent of households where both parents are out of work at least one parent is disabled. There are now more disabled adults living in poverty than either children or pensioners.

Research has estimated that at least 55 per cent of families with disabled children are living in, or at the margins of, poverty. In families with disabled children, 84 per cent of mothers are not working compared with 39 per cent in families with non-disabled children.

It seems the Government listened. In March, Secretary of State for Work and Pensions John Hutton acknowledged that child poverty was 'a disability issue', and that reaching the 2020 target to end all child poverty would demand specific attention to the experiences of families in which someone was disabled.

Income poverty and material deprivation in childhood are unnecessary evils which should be anomalous in any modern, wealthy, civilised society. Child poverty predicts life chances. It damages families, narrows horizons, depresses aspirations and constrains opportunities. It lays waste to human potential and sets in train a lifetime of disadvantage, with enormous costs to both the individuals concerned and to society at large. A child who lives in poverty is less likely to succeed educationally, and more likely to be unemployed and live in poverty when an adult, often setting off the same pattern for their own children. We must break the cycle.

This publication is an extremely timely contribution to that goal. The Treasury recently announced a cross-departmental review concerning disabled children ahead of the 2007 Comprehensive Spending Review. Child poverty is expected to be a key feature. The Department for Work and Pensions (DWP) has just completed consulting on its welfare reform proposals and will be deliberating next steps, critical not just to reducing the numbers on incapacity benefits but to achieving the child poverty targets. The Department for Education and Skills is rolling out the next phases of the *Every Child Matters* strategy, including 'wraparound childcare', extended schools and Sure Start.

Having established that disability needs to be at its heart, what are the particular challenges such a strategy needs to address? We believe they fall into three broad categories:

- Ensuring that measures of poverty and related strategies to deal with it properly account for additional outgoings related to disability.
- Optimising the opportunities for families to establish a living income.
- Identifying and dealing with those environmental, as opposed to intrinsic, factors which give rise to additional outgoings.

Regarding measurement, Tania Burchardt makes an excellent contribution to the debate in this publication. Income is an important, but insufficient, measure of poverty, because both intrinsic and environmental factors shape the ability of different families to achieve equivalent goals with the same amount of money. Research has estimated that on average it costs three times as much to bring up a disabled child as a non-disabled child, and many disabled adults face additional costs in their lives. Therefore, a family in which someone is disabled may have an income of, say, 70 per cent of the mean average (and will therefore not officially be considered to be living in poverty), but will actually be worse off than a family living on an income of 60 per cent of the mean average income but without any disabled family members.

If our real motivation for eradicating child poverty is to promote more equal life chances for all children, our measures need to start by looking at the relative capability of families and disabled children to achieve similar outcomes, not simply at the equivalence of their incomes. Perhaps it could be agreed that the outcomes adopted are those aspirations the Government has set out for all children in the Children Act and *Every Child Matters*. Children should be healthy, safe, make a positive contribution and achieve economic well-being.

The question, then, concerns the substantive inputs different families will require to achieve these outcomes, which by their nature will be different, with some families requiring more than others.

This leads to the second challenge of optimising the opportunities of families to establish a living income. If we accept that disability is associated with extra living costs, then we must also accept that a 'living income' for a family with a disabled member may be higher than for a family without a disabled member. This needs accounting for, both in the degree to which work is made a viable financial option and in defining the point at which public policy can demand the move from benefits to work. We must account for the additional labour market disadvantage faced by disabled people in designing policies and programmes not just to get people into work, but to ensure people can thrive and progress in work. Disabled parents simply getting into and becoming stuck in low-status, low-paid jobs is unlikely to help us achieve our targets. Similarly, we must account for the additional costs and challenges faced by many parents of disabled children in securing appropriate and affordable childcare if work is going to be a viable option for them.

Finally, the link needs to be drawn in public policy between eliminating child poverty and the environmental constraints which create additional costs related to disability, especially if our interest is in promoting more equal life chances. Many families with disabled members face exceptional costs for non-exceptional things, such as childcare, leisure, having a holiday or finding somewhere suitable to live. Many of these costs could be mitigated were disability to be thought about from the start in the design and delivery of services. Perhaps an explicit link could be drawn between measuring the impact of the Disability Discrimination Act, including the recent duty on the public sector to promote equality of opportunity, and eliminating child poverty, with both the Office of Disability Issues in the DWP and the forthcoming Commission for Equality and Human Rights playing a key role. All relevant public policy should perhaps be tested for its impact upon eliminating child poverty.

There is an old African proverb which says 'it takes a village to bring up a child'. Ending child poverty will take the concerted effort of a wide range of players, including those across the Whitehall and Westminster village. This should not be viewed as a burden, but rather as an investment for the future. A problem shared is, of course, a problem halved. This book should be a strong signal to the Government of the commitment and offer of support from a wide range of partners.

Ending child poverty is in this country's interest. Disability is at the heart of the challenge. I commend this book to those serious about rising to it.

Bert Massie
Chair, Disability Rights Commission

Introduction

Gabrielle Preston

The recent publication of the Green Paper on welfare reform, *A New Deal for Welfare: empowering people to work*, and of the *Households Below Average Income* (HBAI) series has moved disability and child poverty up the political agenda. The eagerly (and often anxiously) awaited Green Paper promises to reduce the number of incapacity benefits claimants by one million in the next ten years, while the HBAI figures revealed – disappointingly – that the Government has failed in its pledge to reduce child poverty by a quarter by 2005.[1] To reach the 2010 target – to reduce child poverty by half – a million more children must be lifted out of poverty.[2]

Despite a number of welcome documents and initiatives emanating from the Government, the link between poverty and disability has remained stubbornly in place, and progress on the reduction of child poverty appears to be faltering. Is the Government on the right track with its current policies?

A Route out of Poverty? comprises a short collection of different works, some of which have been written specifically for this publication, some of which draw on submissions issued by CPAG during the course of a protracted consultation process. It considers welfare reform from the perspective of child poverty, and assesses whether current government policies on disabled people and on child poverty complement or detract from each other.

There is, inevitably, significant overlap between the different chapters, and similar themes, arguments and statistical findings thread their way through the book. We hope that these disparate works constitute a cumulative picture, and provide a helpful contextual framework and useful analysis. They raise important questions and pointers for a government that is intent on helping more disabled people move into work, and on moving towards the 2010 target to halve child poverty.

Disability and child poverty

One in three disabled adults of working age are parents,[3] and around a quarter of children living in poverty have a disabled parent.[4] Disability and lone parenthood are also linked. One-quarter of lone parents have a long-standing illness or disability.[5] Two in five children (or 43 per cent) in poverty live in a lone-parent household.[6] It is clearly important to make sure that welfare reform not only assists government initiatives to increase employment for disabled people and lone parents, but that it helps, not hinders, other initiatives to reduce child poverty.

The Government's message

The Government has long argued that disability is both a cause and a consequence of poverty, and that it is committed to breaking the seemingly intractable link between the two. Since 1997 a number of very welcome initiatives have been introduced to help disabled people. Improvements to disability benefits (such as the introduction of the disability premium in tax credits) have been accompanied by initiatives designed to help more disabled people to access work, such as the New Deal for Disabled People and the successful Pathways to Work pilots. The Government's belief that a 'return to work should be a positive and realistic option' and its conviction that 'services should be personalised with a strong focus on delivering support tailored around individual needs'[7] are very welcome.

There is also much to be welcomed in the Green Paper. It recognises the barriers to employment faced by disabled people and lone parents, considers the additional support they need to access jobs, and accepts the importance of providing more adequate financial support to those disabled adults who are unable to work. We endorse the Government's commitment in the foreword 'to ensure that disabled people have the comprehensive civil rights they need' and to reverse 'the inexcusable disadvantage faced by disabled people by delivering substantive equality within a generation.'

But welfare reform has been a long time coming and has been accompanied by mixed messages. On the one hand, the Government has argued (in the words of the then Secretary of State for Work and Pensions, Alan Johnson MP), that:

Our goal is genuine inclusion, stamping out the discrimination and disadvantage that prevents people from fulfilling their potential – and denies society the skills and contributions of those who want to work, but who remain outside the labour market.[8]

On the other hand, the Government has sought to mollify middle England and an often vitriolic press by dismissing the benefit system as 'crackers' (in the words of the subsequent Secretary of State for Work and Pensions, David Blunkett MP) and compounding stigma by stating that working 'will overcome depression and stress a lot more than people sitting at home watching daytime television.'[9]

While some ministers have sought to emphasise that reform of incapacity benefits is designed to liberate disabled people and tap into their skills and capabilities, unhelpful threats of draconian measures have been leaked to the press, including the rumour that £20 would be taken from sick claimants.[10] Alarmist reports about high levels of benefit wastage and fraud[11] appear to have triggered a knee-jerk reaction in a government which is torn between a genuine desire to support disadvantaged and vulnerable groups of people, and a compulsion to be seen as 'tough'.[12]

This somewhat erratic approach is reflected in the Green Paper, which sometimes seems at odds with other government recommendations and policy initiatives such as *Every Child Matters*[13] and the *Child Poverty Review*[14] and fails to give due weight to disabled people's parenting responsibilities, family needs or income adequacy.

There are discrepancies within the Green Paper itself, which we believe reflect wider problems with the Government's policy on disabled people. As CPAG's response to the Green Paper indicates, there has been significantly more research into lone parents than into disabled people.[15] However, despite the parallels – and overlaps – between these two groups, the Green Paper treats them as discrete groups with differing needs, and imposes different levels of conditionality and expectations. It ignores the fact that disabled people are often parents, sometimes lone parents, and that lone parents are often disabled. It is regrettable that the Green Paper has failed to apply lessons learned from the experiences of lone parents to disabled people. We fear that the failure to do so may have a negative impact on child poverty.

The protracted and often hostile debate has engendered high levels of anxiety among disabled people themselves, and scepticism among organisations and individuals who represent them. It has consolidated the impression that the Government is tending to help those who can help themselves, rather than proposing a genuine policy initiative which places the needs of people who are affected by disability at the forefront of reform, and we fear that this may have a negative impact on the implementation of the proposals.

Principles of welfare reform

The underlying ethos of the Government's welfare reform programme, which aims to move one million disabled people off incapacity benefits, 300,000 lone parents into work, and a million older people into employment, is very familiar. Its emphasis is on 'rights and responsibilities', its conviction is that 'too many people had been written off and condemned to a life dependent on benefits', and its belief is that paid employment is 'good for individuals, good for families, good for communities and good for Britain'.

The Green Paper promises to:

- establish a system 'that recognises the **responsibilities** people have to get themselves off benefits, while ensuring that society fulfils its obligations to those unable to help themselves';
- 'build up increased **conditionality** on the basis of what evidence tells us is most effective', but states that 'as support is increased, so will the level of conditionality for claimants';
- '**increase the number of people who leave benefits** quickly to return to work';
- '**reduce much of the complexity surrounding existing benefits** for those facing health problems and disability';
- introduce a '**modernised delivery system** – with the public, private and voluntary sectors working together';
- take steps 'on **prevention and proactive intervention**';
- help 'all low-skilled adults **get the skills they need to succeed in work**' and 'continue our joint working with the UK devolved administrations to support low-skilled adults'.

The main proposal contained in the Green Paper is to replace incapacity benefit (IB) and income support (IS) paid on the grounds of incapacity with a new, contributory and income-related payment (the employment and support allowance), coupled with a requirement to engage in work-focused activities and acquire skills.

But does the approach outlined in the Green Paper address the needs of the UK's most vulnerable groups and are its proposals likely to draw more people out of poverty?

Employment: a route out of poverty?

The Government has long argued that employment is the most effective route out of poverty. Given the stigma that is all too often associated with being on benefits, paid employment can bring significant financial and psychological benefits – including a sense of self-worth and social inclusion. Seventy-seven per cent of children are poor in households in which no adult is in paid work, compared with 3 per cent of children in households with two full-time workers.[16] However, as this book clearly demonstrates, although adequately paid work does lift families out of poverty, and disabled people who are willing and able to work should be assisted to access well-remunerated, sustainable and rewarding jobs, work is by no means the panacea the Government would like it to be. High levels of in-work poverty render employment an unreliable route out of poverty. Over half (54 per cent) of poor children live in a household in which a parent is in work. Twenty-nine per cent of children living with a lone parent who works full time fall in the bottom two-fifths of the income distribution, and this rises to 58 per cent for lone parents who work part time.[17]

High levels of in-work poverty are a particular source of concern as the Government begins to target more disadvantaged groups that are furthest from the labour market.

Furthermore, there are doubts about whether the Government's ambitious employment targets are realistic. One Parent Families reports that the Government's desire to move 300,000 lone parents into work is extremely ambitious as it requires lone parent employment to rise over the next five years 'three times as fast as it did in the last five.'[18] Researchers confirm that increasing the employment rate further is likely to become more difficult because lone parents who remain outside employment are 'increasingly less well skilled and concentrated in rented housing, and are a group for whom work incentives remain weak.'[19] Lone parents are more likely to access part-time, low-paid employment, and currently work may not prove an effective route out of poverty for them. We fear that the same holds true for disabled people, particularly if they are parents. This publication raises serious concerns about focusing solely on employment as a route out of poverty.

Barriers to employment

Although the Green Paper highlights 'discrimination, policy design and delivery, physical and environmental barriers, and a lack of empowerment' and reports that 'the Government and external stakeholders must act to provide additional help and support so that people can fulfil their potential', it also calls for:

> ...a clear response from individual citizens themselves: they need to meet their responsibility to take the necessary steps to re-enter the labour market when they have a level of capacity and capability that makes this possible.

However, *A Route out of Poverty?* reveals that disabled parents – many of whom are lone parents, some of whom also have disabled children – continue to face sometimes insurmountable hurdles to employment because poor service provision compounds the difficulties they experience balancing their health conditions alongside their parenting responsibilities.

Furthermore, despite the extension of the Disability Discrimination Act, discrimination in society as a whole – and in the workplace in particular – renders employment extremely difficult for some disabled people, particularly if they have mental health problems, learning disabilities or fluctuating conditions. We are also concerned that the emphasis on work as the only worthwhile and appropriate route out of poverty risks perpetuating a negative image of benefit recipients, which will do little to redress – and may increase – the high levels of discrimination at work and in society as a whole.

Given the structural barriers to employment faced by disabled parents, many of which are not within their power to resolve (such as problems with childcare or transport, poor education, training or skills, or the lack of suitable, local jobs) this book questions whether it is just to expect all parents to engage in work-focused activities with the expectation that they access employment.

In-work poverty

As illustrated throughout this book, even if the Government is successful in drawing more disabled people into employment, there are doubts about whether paid employment will prove to be an effective route out of poverty for a group of people who are more likely to move into low-paid, low-skilled jobs, and for whom salaries may not cover additional costs.

Despite the very positive approach adopted towards employment in the Green Paper, *A Route out of Poverty?* raises concerns about whether it is right to expect people to look for jobs that may not exist, or to encourage people to move into unreliable, poor quality jobs that may have a negative impact upon parents' and children's lives, and leave them living in poverty. Research on lone parents undertaken for the Department for Work and Pensions (DWP) concludes that supporting lone parents to access sustainable, well-paid jobs is more important than compelling lone parents who are furthest from the labour market to attend work-focused interviews. We believe this statement also holds true for sick or disabled parents.[20] There are also concerns that increasing employment among those least able to sustain it may increase the 'churn' rate between benefits and employment.[21]

Benefits

Access and adequacy

The Green Paper states that 'there is a clear link between benefits dependency and hardship.' And yet it is the Government that has set 'safety net' benefits, such as IS and jobseeker's allowance (JSA), well below the poverty line. This book highlights the fact that ensuring disabled adults and children receive the disability benefits to which they are entitled is essential to safeguard families from poverty, and may result in an improvement in health. However, disability benefits, such as disability living allowance, and premiums within IS and tax credits that provide much needed additional financial support for disabled people, are poorly advertised, hard to access without the support of a welfare rights specialist, and erratically administered.

Research indicates that moving in and out of employment, and on and off benefits, renders parents and their children vulnerable to severe and persistent poverty. An influential report on children who experience poverty emphasises that:

> Policy must recognise that work is not possible for all parents at all times [and] benefits must be adequate to protect children from poverty at times when work is not an option...[22]

Although the Green Paper recognises the importance of 'making it easier for people to return to their previous benefit levels' if employment does not work out, and has put a number of options in place 'for people to try out work before leaving incapacity benefit' (such as engaging in unlimited voluntary work and various forms of part-time paid work), it does not engage with benefit adequacy. Ongoing administrative problems within the benefit and tax credit systems, which are administered by different government departments, undermine the effective implementation of linking rules and this generates financial insecurity for families who move in and out of work.

To improve both child and parental employment outcomes, parents – and their children – should be supported irrespective of their work status. The Government's refusal to accede to repeated calls for a review of the adult rates of IS and JSA and for a general review of benefit adequacy continues to generate disquiet among poverty commentators.[23]

Rights and responsibilities

Much is made in the Green Paper about rights and responsibilities, and many government initiatives emphasise the importance of choice. However, we are concerned that the increase in responsibilities for some of the most vulnerable groups saps both their choice and their rights. Furthermore, responsibilities appear to be disproportionately placed on individuals who have fewer rights and less power.

For example, although the Green Paper reports that 'the current system fails to engage with employers or to use them to channel more and better jobs towards disadvantaged people', the reality is that disabled people themselves are landed with the responsibility to find jobs, while employers (some of whom show scant regard for the Disability Discrimination Act or flexible family-friendly policies) are not being required to ensure that appropriate, sustainable and well-paid jobs are available.

Despite legislation, work routines and structures are often not sufficiently flexible to enable either lone parents or disabled people to work.

Furthermore, as the Green Paper acknowledges, the Government has the responsibility to ensure that appropriate support services are put in place to support sick or disabled people irrespective of whether they are in work or not. And yet, a recent report indicates a woeful lack of support for people suffering from mental health problems or depression, who account for the largest group of people on IB.[24]

International evidence

The Government, which is keen to learn from the experiences of other countries, needs to take account of lessons emanating from the US where 'time limit and work requirement provisions prompted a shift from an ongoing cash assistance system to one focused on moving parents into permanent jobs' under the Temporary Assistance for Needy Family (TANF) programme. The efficacy of such an approach is by no means clear. Although TANF has resulted 'in a significant growth in employment among lone-parent families' – from 57 per cent in 1994 to 70 per cent in 2000 – data suggests that 'earnings remained low for most of the affected families...[and] annual earnings did not come close to the poverty line for a family of three.'[25]

Although in the UK, welfare reform does not appear to be driven (as it does in the US)[26] by a desire simply to reduce benefit caseload, we are concerned that a number of proposals, such as measures 'to reward primary care staff who take steps to support individuals to remain in or return to work' may be misconstrued (not least by staff administering the new system) as a drive to reduce the benefit caseload. Should the desire to reduce the number of people on benefits take precedence over improving the quality of jobs, it will do nothing to tackle child poverty.

Research undertaken for the DWP argues that:

> If the goal of policymakers is both to promote employment and reduce child poverty, there is a need to do far more than the US has done to date in addressing skill-building, employment retention and advancement, and in broadening the availability of work supports for low-earning families.[27]

For the moment, however, it is not clear that the Green Paper proposals are sufficient or resources adequate to put such a strategy in place.

Increased compulsion

This book highlights a number of concerns about the increase in conditionality, and the introduction of benefit sanctions for sick or disabled people who do not engage in work-focused activities. An increase in mandatory work-focused interviews and the imposition of financial sanctions, whether by statutory, voluntary or – even more worrying – private sector providers, will be costly for individuals and government alike. Using voluntary sector organisations which currently represent the needs of sick or disabled people to police the new system will undermine a valuable and independent source of support for disabled people.

The Green Paper states that 'we will wish to build up increased conditionality on the basis of what evidence tells us is most effective' and yet the Government appears to be ignoring evidence from its successful pilot schemes (Pathways to Work and the New Deal). Despite, or perhaps because of, the voluntary element within both schemes, they have succeeded in increasing the employment rate for disabled people and lone parents. The Pathways to Work evaluation and the Government itself emphasise that one of the strengths of the pilots is the high level of interest it generated despite the lack of compulsion.[28] The *Pre-Budget Report 2004* confirms that:

> The pilots are also generating significant interest from existing IB claimants in the pilot district, who are currently not required to take part in the programme.[29]

The same is true for the New Deal for Lone Parents[30] which, according to the DWP, has been 'popular with participants [and] been a successful and cost-effective programme that significantly increased the chances of participants to enter work.'[31] Given the success of these programmes, it is hard to know why the Government is keen to increase conditionality, particularly as this is likely to have a negative impact on the most vulnerable groups.

The Green Paper accepts that:

> International evidence shows that stricter conditionality can have a very limited benefit if it is applied without childcare support and incentives to work. Stronger requirements can be crucial in getting lone parents off benefits, but the macroeconomic environment is a key determinant of their participation in the labour market.

A recent increase in unemployment, which has disproportionately affected women workers, raises concerns about the capacity of the labour market.

Services

The provision of joined-up, accessible and appropriate support services is at the heart of the Government's strategy on the eradication of child poverty. The implementation of the Disability Discrimination Act and the very welcome publication of *Improving the Life Chances of Disabled People*[33] illustrate that the Government recognises that it is the responsibility of a wide range of government departments to address the needs of disabled people. However, we are concerned that the Green Paper does not reflect this inter-departmental perspective and, indeed, ignores a number of initiatives emanating from other departments.

The success of welfare reform is dependent on the provision of effective and joined-up services, but there are concerns that current provision is not sufficiently flexible and resourced to provide the support needed to help more disabled people access work. Although the Green Paper cites *Improving the Life Chances of Disabled People* and highlights the creation of a new cross-government Office for Disability Issues, the programme of welfare reform sometimes seems at odds with these and other policy initiatives.

Although the Government accepts that disabled people with parenting and caring responsibilities face particular barriers to employment, and statistics indicate that children who live with one or more disabled adult face a disproportionate risk of living in poverty, their particular needs have not been directly addressed within the Green Paper. There is little or no recognition of disabled people's parenting or caring responsibilities in the section on helping ill or disabled people. While the Green Paper refers to the Department of Health's Green Paper *Independence, Well-being and Choice*, the proposals do not appear to have been informed by other government documents, which emphasise that parental responsibilities must be taken into consideration when assessing a disabled adult's care needs. For example, a recent report published by the Department of Health stresses that:

> In the course of assessing an individual's needs, councils should recognise that adults, who have parenting responsibilities for a child under 18 years, may require help with these responsibilities.

Multiple disadvantage

The Government has identified a number of disadvantages that place children at risk of poor outcomes, including poor housing, poor schools and poor services. It has also identified a number of groups as being at particular risk of poverty, including some families from black and minority ethnic backgrounds, families with three or more children and families with disabled children. However, the Green Paper does not address the fact that many disabled and lone parents fall into some – or all – of the groups identified by the Government as being disadvantaged.

Support for Parents: the best start for children has identified disabled children and children with special educational needs as being at particular risk.[35] Many children who fall into these groups live in disabled or lone-parent families. Although the Green Paper emphasises that *Improving the Life Chances of Disabled People* included measures 'on improving support for families with young disabled childen' and 'helping a smooth transition into adulthood by, for example, removing 'cliff edges' in service provision', the increase in conditionality may result in welfare reform undermining other initiatives to support these groups of children and young people.

We are particularly concerned about the possible impact the new proposals will have on young disabled people, many of whom are care leavers. *Support for Parents: the best start for children* focuses on the needs of children in care, reporting that they are:

> …likely to be poor by the time they enter care…are seven times more likely than the wider population to suffer from mental health problems [and] have poor educational outcomes.[36]

Welfare reform should support and not penalise this vulnerable group of young people.

Prevention

Although the Government accepts that disability is a cause of poverty, much less is made of the fact that living on a low income *increases* the risk of disability, although this is borne out by significant research on health inequalities.[37] A recent report confirms that:

The onset of disability is by no means a random occurrence. On the contrary, those who are already disadvantaged are already at significantly greater risk of becoming disabled.[38]

Although a number of interlinking factors increase the likelihood of becoming disabled, including having low or no educational qualifications and being out of work, research identifies 'a close association between low household income and a high risk of becoming disabled across all age groups.'[39] Furthermore, living on a low income not only increases the likelihood of becoming sick and disabled, but the average household income of those who become disabled is already falling prior to the onset of disability.[40] It is not just low income that generates stress and ill-health, high levels of inequality take their toll on the health of the nation. Recent research highlights poorer health in countries with high levels of inequality.[41]

However, although the Government accepts that 'more needs to be done to address these reinforcing cycles of underperformance and deprivation' and confirms that 'a significant proportion of new claimants come onto incapacity benefits from employment', the focus in the Green Paper appears to be more on preventing ill-health in the workplace than avoiding the sort of poverty that is so closely associated with disability and ill-health.[42]

While we agree that more should be done to ensure that employers provide a safe and healthy working environment that supports all disabled people and avoids the onset of sickness or ill-health, we believe that considerations of income adequacy – whether a person is on benefit or in paid employment – are essential to avoid the sort of inter-generational disadvantage that is all too often generated by disability and ill-health. Strenuous efforts are needed to ensure that disabled adults, children and young people are able to access the financial, educational, health and support services they need, irrespective of their work status.

Deserving or undeserving?

There is a worrying element of division within the Government's programme of welfare reform between those viewed as deserving and those perhaps as less deserving of financial support. On the one hand, the Green Paper reports that:

> For those claimants with the most severe health conditions or disabilities, the benefit will be paid without benefit conditionality and they should get more money than they do now.

On the other hand, it threatens to reduce benefit:

> …in a series of slices, ultimately to the level of jobseeker's allowance if recipients of the employment component fail to undertake work-related interviews, agree an action plan and, 'as resources allow', participate.

While disabled parents and disabled young people will be placed on a 'basic allowance' set at JSA rates, the Government has clearly stated that lone parents will not be subjected to 'an unrestricted requirement to search for work' and that moving them from IS onto JSA would be 'expensive, unfair and ineffectual.'[43] It is important that an invidious element of divide and rule does not creep into the Government's programme of welfare reform.

However, the focus on benefit fraud risks doing just that. Although the Green Paper reports that 'it is estimated that around 1.2 per cent of expenditure on incapacity benefits is overpaid through fraud and error – this is one of the lowest rates for the benefits system', it then sets out detailed information about how it will deal with fraud. Random, 'ad hoc checks to be carried out by a dedicated team which will be specially created for this purpose' to 'provide confirmation to the genuine claimant of the appropriateness and correctness of their ongoing entitlement and also assurance to the taxpayer of the integrity and security of the benefit' will do little to dispel myths about fraud. Far from reassuring tax payers and members of the public that the DWP is being vigilant, this focus risks compounding the view that recipients of disability benefits are often fraudulent.

Outline of *A Route out of Poverty?*

The first section of this book provides a general framework. In **Chapter 1**, Guy Palmer considers the different ways in which disabled people are disadvantaged within the labour market. He discusses poverty rates among disabled people, reviews how these have changed over time and compares them with the equivalent rate for non-disabled people. He considers the relationship between poverty and work, and discusses why so many disabled people are not in employment. He highlights some shocking statistics about the difficulties disabled people experience accessing work irrespective of their level of qualifications, and emphasises that even if the Government is successful in its aim to help move people into employment, there will always be many disabled people reliant on benefits, and that benefit adequacy must be an integral part of welfare reform.

In **Chapter 2**, we reproduce an article by Richard Olsen and Hugh Stickland that first appeared in *At Greatest Risk: the children most likely to be poor*, published by CPAG in 2005, highlighting the situation for disabled parents. Using data from a variety of sources, they expose the strong association between child poverty and parental worklessness, and the close connection between disability and unemployment. They ask why, given the Government's commitment to reduce child poverty and its determination to draw disabled people off IB into work, 'there are no goals, targets, interventions or programmes specifically tailored for disabled parents?'

In **Chapter 3**, Tania Burchardt considers child poverty in families with disabled parents or disabled children and young people. Although statistics on disability and poverty are stark, this chapter emphasises that they underestimate the real incidence of poverty in households affected by disability because they include benefit income designed to meet extra costs (such as disability living allowance), but ignore the extra costs they are designed to meet. The author questions whether the employment opportunities exist, particularly for young people, to meet the Government's target to get disabled adults into work.

In **Chapter 4**, Gabrielle Preston considers how the proposals in the Green Paper will affect disabled parents. Based on interviews with a small number of sick or disabled parents, it describes their attitudes to and experiences of paid employment, the accessibility and adequacy of disability benefits (including IB), the availability and appropriateness of services, and the impact that government policy has had on their children's lives. The interviews reveal ongoing problems with discrimination and highlight the failure of the Government to communicate its message on employment effectively or sensitively to those affected.

Chapter 5 is an edited and updated version of CPAG's submissions to the Work and Pensions Select Committee inquiry into Pathways to Work, the reform of IB, and the Green Paper itself.

Finally, in the **Conclusion** we raise a number of specific issues about the Green Paper and its implementation, and provide some clear messages for the Government.

Notes

1   In March 1997, the year that New Labour came to power, 4.2 million (or a shocking one in four) children in Great Britain lived in poverty. In March 1999, Prime Minister Tony Blair delivered New Labour's ambitious pledge to eradicate child poverty by 2020. A number of challenging targets were promised en route to abolition: child poverty would be reduced by a quarter by 2005 (down to 3.1 million children) and by half by 2010 (down to 2.1 million).

2   See M Brewer, A Goodman, J Shaw and L Sibieta, *Poverty and Inequality in Britain*, Institute for Fiscal Studies, 2006, which reports that 'reducing child poverty by 1 million between 2004/05 and 2010/11 to meet the target is likely to require significant new spending measures.' (p57)

3   See H Stickland, Background paper for the HMT/DWP seminar 'Disabled Parents and Employment', 24 November 2003

4   Department for Work and Pensions, *Households Below Average Income 1994/95-2004/05*, Corporate Document Services, 2006, indicates that after housing costs have been accounted for, 24 per cent of the 3.4 million poor children in Great Britain (around 816,000) lived with one or more disabled adult in 2004/05. The risk of income poverty for this group was 40 per cent (against an average risk for all children of 27 per cent).

5   One Parent Families, *Meeting the Target: how can the Government achieve a 70 per cent employment rate for lone parents?* One Parent Families, 2005

6   See note 4, Table 4.4

7   Cabinet Office, Prime Minister's Strategy Unit, *Improving the Life Chances of Disabled People*, 2005 (a joint report with the Department for Work and Pensions, Department of Health, Department for Education and Skills and Office of the Deputy Prime Minister)

8   Speech to the Institute for Public Policy Research seminar, 'Fit for Purpose: welfare to work and incapacity benefit', 7 February 2005, available at www.dwp.gov.uk/aboutus/2005/07_02_05_ippr.asp

9   'Work and Pensions Secretary, David Blunkett, said that a strategy would be unveiled later this week to tackle welfare fraud' in scotsman.com news, 11 October 2005

10 See P Toynbee, 'No More Talk of Scroungers: it's a victory for civilisation' in The *Guardian*, 10 January 2006: '...the threat to cut £20 a week from sick claimants, as suggested by No.10 in a leaked letter, has been sent back to the asylum it came from.'

11 House of Commons Committee of Public Accounts, *Fraud and Error in Benefit Expenditure, Fourth Report of Session 2005/06*, October 2005, reports that 'in 2003/04 the DWP lost an estimated...£2 billion of fraud and £1 billion of customer and official error' and that 'the recent major reorganisation to form

Jobcentre Plus and the Pension Service led to an increase in the level of errors by officials.' Its recently published *Tackling the Complexity of the Benefits System, Thirty-sixth Report of Session 2005/06* confirms 'high levels of error by staff and customers' and that 'fraud in key benefits has reduced since 1997/98, but levels of error have increased recently, in part because of organisational change within the Department'.

12 See www.direct.gov.uk: 'Campaign Gives Tough Warning to Benefit Cheats': 'Anti-fraud Minister Malcolm Wicks...urged the public to support the campaign by reporting people who are committing benefit fraud.' Available at www.pm.gov.uk/output/page3799.asp

13 *Every Child Matters: change for children*, was delivered by ministers responsible for delivering services for children and young people at the Department for Education and Skills, Department of Health, Department for Work and Pensions, HM Treasury, Office of the Deputy Prime Minister, Department for Environment, Food and Rural Affairs, Department of Trade and Industry, Ministry of Defence, Department for Constitutional Affairs, Home Office, and Department for Culture, Media and Sport

14 HM Treasury, *Child Poverty Review*, The Stationery Office, 2004

15 Child Poverty Action Group, *Response to Department for Work and Pensions' Green Paper: A New Deal for Welfare: empowering people to work*, April 2006, available at www.cpag.org.uk

16 P Dornan 'Working a Way Out of Poverty?' in G Preston (ed), *At Greatest Risk: the children most likely to be poor*, CPAG, 2005

17 Department for Work and Pensions, *Households Below Average Income 1994/95-2003/04*, Corporate Document Services, 2005

18 See One Parent Families briefing for Westminster Hall debate on lone parent employment, 2 March 2006.

19 P Gregg and S Harkness, *Welfare Reform and Lone Parents in the UK*, CMPO Working Paper 03/72, June 2003

20 M Evans, S Harkness and R Ortiz, *Lone Parents Cycling Between Work and Benefits*, DWP Research Report 217, Corporate Document Services, 2004

21 See note 20. The authors report that, while the employment rate for lone parents has increased and the number of lone parents leaving jobs has fallen, the rate of job exit is considerably higher for lone parents than for other groups, even after personal and job characteristics are controlled for.

22 See L Adelman, S Middleton and K Ashworth, *Britain's Poorest Children: severe and persistent poverty and social exclusion*, Save the Children, 2003

23 See, for example, R Lister 'Poverty: the case for a review of benefit levels' in *Compass Thinkpiece 5*, Compass, 2006

24 See S Boseley, 'Depression is UK's Biggest Social Problem, Government Told' in the *Guardian*, 28 April 2006. Reporting on an article by Richard Layard, emeritus professor at the Centre for Economic Performance at the London School of Economics in the *British Medical Journal*, the *Guardian* reports that 15 per cent of the British population is suffering from depression and anxiety disorders, of whom only 4 per cent received psychological therapies in the last year. One million people on incapacity benefit suffer from a mental illness – more than the number of unemployed.

25 See J Millar and M Evans (eds), *Lone Parents and Employment: international comparisons of what works*, Centre for the Analysis of Social Policy, 2003. The authors report that the 'shift from a focus on income maintenance to a focus on job placement and employment preparation' is driven primarily by the desire for 'caseload reduction.' (p45)

26 See note 25

27 See note 25

28 See B Blythe, *Incapacity Benefit Reforms: Pathways to Work pilots' performance and analysis*, DWP Working Paper 26, 2006. The author states 'There were a total of 147,950 starts to the Pathways to Work process…11,200 are currently identifiable as voluntary participants' (7.6 per cent). 'There were a total of 19,550 Pathways job entries to end of August…3,010 were from the voluntary customer group' (15.5 per cent). 'This means that jobs from voluntary customers are making a significant contribution to Pathways performance'. (pp11 and 16)

29 HM Treasury, *Pre-Budget Report*, 2004, p77

30 Department for Work and Pensions, *Opportunity for All: seventh annual report*, The Stationery Office, 2005, reports that the New Deal for Lone Parents is 'a voluntary programme available to all non-employed lone parents, and has a strong focus on providing lone parents with work-focused information and advice, particularly in relation to the financial implications of employment'. It has been 'popular with participants [and] been a successful and cost-effective programme that significantly increased the chances of participants to enter work.' (p48)

31 See note 25

32 L Elliott, 'Unemployment Heads for 1m by Summer' in the *Guardian*, 13 April 2006. The *Guardian* reports that 'the slowdown in consumer spending is taking a particular toll on female jobs in the service sector.'

33 See note 7

34 Department of Health, *Fair Access to Care Services: guidance on eligibility criteria for adult social care*, 2003, p2

35 HM Treasury and Department for Education and Skills, *Support for Parents: the best start for children*, The Stationery Office, 2005

36 See note 35

37 See J Carvel, 'Wealth Brings 17 More Years of Health' in the *Guardian*, 25 February 2005. Discussing findings from a recent report from the Office for National Statistics, *The Guardian* reports a poorer man's healthy life expectancy is only 49.4 years, nearly 17 years less than a man from a prosperous ward, and a woman's healthy life expectancy is 51.7 in deprived wards and 68.5 years in the most prosperous wards.

38 T Burchardt, *Being and Becoming: social exclusion and the onset of disability*, CASEreport 21, Centre for Analysis of Social Exclusion, 2003, p1

39 See note 38, pp22-23

40 S Jenkins and J Rigg, *Disability and Disadvantage: selection, onset and duration effects*, CASEpaper74, Centre for Analysis of Social Exclusion, 2003

41 See P Toynbee, 'Inequality Kills' in the *Guardian*, 30 July 2005. Reviewing Professor Richard Wilkinson's book, *The Impact of Inequality: how to make sick societies healthier*, Routledge, 2005, she comments that 'social status and respect matter beyond anything, and the psychological damage done by being at the bottom is crippling.'

42 For example, the Green Paper reports 'Our first priority must be to reduce the likelihood of people developing health problems that may result in them having to give up work and becoming dependent on benefits. Where they do develop health problems, we want to help them manage these so that they can remain in work and achieve their potential.' (p29)

43 Department for Work and Pensions, *Five Year Strategy: opportunity and security throughout life*, The Stationery Office, 2005, p38

One

Disabled people, poverty and the labour market

Guy Palmer

Introduction

Thirty per cent of disabled adults of working age (aged 25 to retirement) are living in poverty – around one and a half million people. This poverty rate is around double that for non-disabled adults and, unlike that for children and pensioners, rather than having fallen in recent years, is arguably rising.

The Government's anti-poverty strategy is centred on the phrase 'work for those who can, security for those who cannot'. For disabled working-age adults, neither part of this phrase is yet in place.

- **'Work for those who can.'** Sixty per cent of disabled adults want to work, but only 40 per cent are currently working. The other 20 per cent – one million people – are effectively saying that they have not been able to find a job.
- **'Security for those who cannot.'** Half of disabled adults living in workless households are also living in poverty. This is, again, around one million people. For these people, the social security benefits they receive are not sufficient to lift them out of poverty.

Disability and its measures

There is no standard way of deciding whether or not someone is disabled and different surveys use somewhat different definitions. In broad terms, however, there are three types of method.[1]

- The most widely used, single-item survey instrument for assessing activity limitation is the **self-reported limiting long-standing illness or disability question**. Variations of this question intend to capture the perceived disabling effects of chronic ill-health, and physical and sensory impairments.
- The second type of measure aims to assess **work-limiting disability**, as defined by the respondent's perceptions of the restriction in her or his capacity for paid work.
- The final type of measure seeks to identify whether respondents have a **disability covered by the Disability Discrimination Act 1995**. This defines disability as a 'physical or mental impairment which has a substantial and long-term adverse effect on his ability to carry out normal day-to-day activities.'

Although these methods are all rather different, they have several features in common, namely:

- They all estimate that there are around five million adults aged 25 to retirement who are disabled.
- They all use a definition that covers disability arising from mental health as well as from physical health.
- They all show that there are substantial numbers of younger adults who are disabled.

These points are important because they counter the popular misconception in the public's mind that the word 'disability' means either 'people in wheelchairs' or 'older men with bad backs'. In fact, two-fifths of claimants of incapacity benefit (IB) have 'mental and behavioural disorders' compared with one-fifth who have 'muscular-skeletal disorders.'[2] Two-fifths are aged under 45.

Poverty among disabled working-age adults

Thirty per cent of disabled adults aged 25 to retirement are living in poverty.[3] This is around one and a half million people. Figure 1.1 shows how this rate has changed over time and how it compares with the poverty rate for non-disabled adults. There are three messages, all sombre.

- The 30 per cent poverty rate for disabled working-age adults is twice that of their non-disabled counterparts.
- While little significance can be attached to year-to-year movements, the poverty rate for disabled working-age adults is now somewhat higher than it was during the mid- and late-1990s.
- The amount by which the disabled poverty rate exceeds the non-disabled poverty rate is now markedly higher than it was in the 1990s.

Figure 1.1
Poverty rates for disabled and non-disabled adults

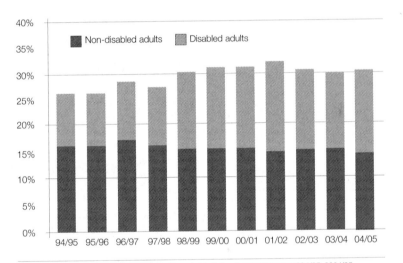

Source: Department for Work and Pensions, *Households Below Average Income 1994/95–2004/05*, Corporate Document Services, 2006

Furthermore, around two-fifths of the disabled working-age people in poverty are single adults without dependent children. As such, many may lack day-to-day company and support, leading to social exclusion as well as poverty.

The lack of progress in reducing poverty rates among disabled people contrasts with the falling poverty rates for those two groups which have been the target of the Government's anti-poverty strategy in recent years, namely children and pensioners. As a result, a higher proportion of disabled working-age people now live in poverty than either children or pensioners.

The relationship between poverty and work

Figure 1.2 shows the how the risk of a person with a work-limiting disability being in poverty varies by the work status of the household. 'All working' is where one adult is in full-time work and the other (if applicable) in full-time or part-time work; 'some working' is where no one is working full time, but one or more are working part time; and 'none working' is where none of the adults in the household are working. It shows the following:

- Unsurprisingly, work substantially reduces the risk of being in poverty. Less than 5 per cent of disabled people in 'all working' households are in poverty compared with 55 per cent of those in workless households.
- Social security benefits are clearly insufficient to bring many disabled workless households out of poverty. Furthermore, unlike those for children and pensioners, the levels of benefits for disabled people have essentially been restricted to inflation-only rises since 1997 and have, therefore, fallen behind average incomes.

Figure 1.2

Poverty rates for disabled people by household work status

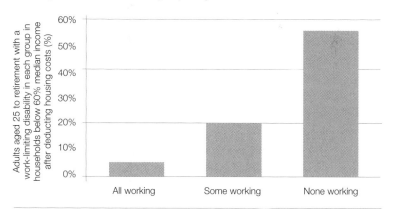

Source: Department for Work and Pensions, *Households Below Average Income 1994/95–2004/05*, Corporate Document Services, 2006; the data is the average for the years 2002/03 to 2004/05

The main reason why the poverty rate for disabled people is so high is that relatively few disabled people work: 60 per cent of adults aged 25 to retirement with a work-limiting disability are currently not working compared with only 15 per cent of their non-disabled counterparts. However, many of those who are not working say that they want to work, but have not been able to find a job: 20 per cent of disabled adults aged 25 to retirement – one million people – are not working, but say they want to.

Figure 1.3 shows how this rate has changed over time and how it compares with the equivalent rate for non-disabled adults. It shows the following:

- The vast majority of disabled adults who are not working but want to count as 'economically inactive' rather than 'unemployed'. This is because, although they want to work, they fail to meet one of the two criteria required to be considered 'unemployed' – namely, that they are available to start work in the next two weeks and have been actively seeking work in the last four weeks.
- The proportion of people with a work-limiting disability who lack, but want, work has declined from 25 per cent to 19 per cent over the last six years, while the comparable rate for people without such a disability has declined from 7 per cent to 5 per cent. In both cases, these 'want work' rates have declined by a quarter. This shows that there has not been any tardiness on the part of disabled, working-age adults to respond to the better employment conditions of recent years.

Even if all those wanting work found it, the employment rate for disabled people would still only be 60 per cent (the 40 per cent who are currently working plus the 20 per cent who say they want to). This means that there will always be many disabled people reliant on benefits.

The conclusion from this analysis is that the problem disabled people face is the result neither of a generous benefits regime that offers disabled people a 'comfortable' existence, nor of a failure on the part of disabled people to respond to the overall growth in jobs. Rather, it is because, despite the improved economic situation and the desire to work, many people have not been able to find jobs. In a situation in which one-fifth of people with a work-limiting disability still lack but want work, reform of the way in which the Department for Work and Pensions supports these people is clearly important.

Figure 1.3

'Lacking but wanting work' rates for disabled and non-disabled people

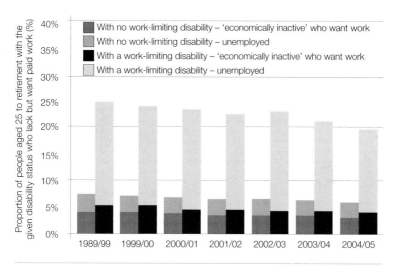

Source: *Labour Force Survey*, National Statistics/Palgrave Macmillan, 2004; the data is for the four quarters to winter 2004/05

Why do so many disabled people want, but lack, work?

One possibility is that it is not disability *per se* that is to blame, but the fact that disabled people have fewer qualifications. Certainly, the lower a person's level of qualifications, the higher the risk that they will find themselves lacking, but wanting, work. However, as Figure 1.4 shows, at every level of qualification, a disabled person is much more likely than a non-disabled person to be lacking, but wanting, work – to such an extent that a disabled person with a degree is more likely than a non-disabled person with no qualifications to find her/himself lacking, but wanting, work. With a pattern this clear cut, higher 'lacking but wanting work' rates cannot simply be explained away by lower qualifications.

Figure 1.4

'Lacking but wanting work' rates by level of qualification

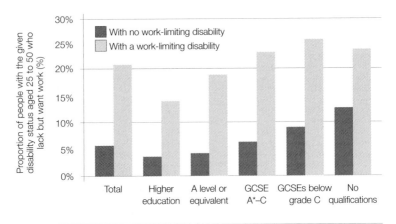

Source: *Labour Force Survey*, National Statistics/Palgrave Macmillan, 2004; the data is for the four quarters to winter 2004/05

Not only do disabled people face a much higher risk of being out of work, they are also somewhat more likely to be low paid than non-disabled colleagues with similar qualifications (Figure 1.5).[4]

Similarly, disabled full-time male workers, full-time female workers and part-time workers are all somewhat more likely to be low paid than their non-disabled counterparts.

The finding that, at every level of qualification, people with a work-limiting disability are more likely to be low paid and more likely to be 'lacking but wanting work' than people without a disability is of great importance. According to basic economic theory, such a situation cannot arise simply as a result of disabled people being more reluctant than non-disabled people to take particular jobs at particular rates of pay. Rather, it is only possible if the labour market is effectively discriminating against them.

'Discrimination' is a sensitive word and it is important to stress that the outcome observed is 'after the event' – that is, the sum total of the effects of all employment decisions taken by all employers. It comes about despite, no doubt, many employers' good intentions. Rather than overt discrimination, it probably arises through a mixture of risk-averseness (for example, small companies not wanting to take a risk by employing dis-

Figure 1.5

Risk of low pay by level of qualification

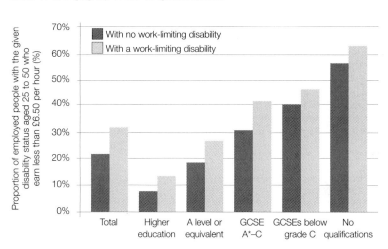

Source: *Labour Force Survey*, National Statistics/Palgrave Macmillan, 2004; the data is for the four quarters to winter 2004/05

abled people) and ignorance (for example, about what disabled people can do, how the Government's Access to Work initiative can support disabled people in work, etc). There are also other factors – for example, problems with transport to and from work, that are the fault of neither the would-be employee nor the would-be employer.

Nevertheless, government reports refer to 'attitude' problems on the part of employers.[5] Also, the recommendations for remedial action from the Prime Minister's Strategy Unit include employer-led campaigns to promote the business benefits of employing disabled people, establishing a single point of information for employers and developing a new system of accreditation for employers. When considering benefit reforms then, it is right to use the word 'discrimination' because it reminds policy makers that, whatever the intentions, it is the reality faced by disabled people.

Three specific conclusions can be drawn from the evidence of discrimination:

- First, while discrimination persists, the goal of substantially increasing the rate of employment among disabled people can only, in practice,

Figure 1.6

Risk of low pay by full-/part-time and gender

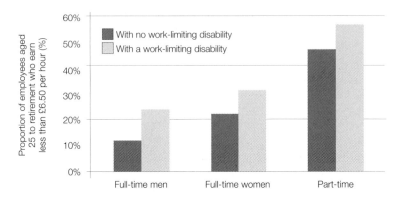

Source: *Labour Force Survey*, National Statistics/Palgrave Macmillan, 2004; the data is the average for the years 2001/02 to 2003/04

be realised at the expense of lowering even further the average earnings of disabled people.

- Second, since changing employer attitudes is bound to take a long time, benefit reform needs to be implemented on the clear understanding that big shifts in employment will also take a long time.

- Third, the Government needs to follow through on the observation in its five-year strategy about the 'need to change the expectations and attitudes of…employers'.[6] By doing so, it would gain a better understanding of the whole problem, with consequent improvements to benefit reform itself.

Conclusion: what should be the goals of reform?

A major objective of the Government's plan to reform IB is to help one million disabled people to get a job. This objective is a good one, but it will only be successful if it tackles the discrimination against disabled people that effectively operates in the labour market. Any reform that exclusively concentrates on disabled would-be workers while ignoring employers reflects an incomplete understanding of the problem.

Even if employment rates among disabled people start rising rapidly, many disabled people will remain dependent on social security benefits for the foreseeable future. But, unlike benefits for children and pensioners, the level of benefits for disabled people have essentially been restricted to inflation-only rises since 1997 and have, therefore, fallen behind average incomes. The long-neglected question of the level of these benefits must, therefore, be addressed.

The high proportion of disabled people who lack, but want, work confirms the rightness of setting higher employment for disabled people as one of the Government's goals. But the high levels of poverty among disabled people, coupled with the difficulties presented by the labour market, show that the problem cannot be tackled through benefit reform alone. Rather, a much more balanced approach is needed and the question is how to stimulate it. One possibility would be for IB reforms to be designed with three, rather than just one, goal in mind:

- a higher employment rate for disabled people;
- a poverty rate no higher than for non-disabled people; *and*
- an end to the 'disability pay gap'.

Developing policy within this framework might be more complex, but to ignore this complexity, as the Government is in danger of doing at the moment with its single-minded pursuit of the employment target, risks failure in this area and a deepening of problems in others.

Notes

1   These definitions are drawn from M Bajekal, T Harries, R Breman and K Wood-field, *Review of Disability Estimates and Definitions*, Department for Work and Pensions, 2004

2   Department for Work and Pensions, *Incapacity Benefit and Severe Disablement Allowance Quarterly Summary Statistics*, February 2005, Table IB1.5

3   This is using the main measure of income poverty used by the Government and others, namely a household income that is 60 per cent or less of the average (median) household income in that year. This draws on the data that was available for 2004/05. In that year, the 60 per cent threshold was worth £183 per week for a two-adult household, £100 per week for a single adult, £260 per week for two adults living with two children and £186 per week for a single adult living with two children. This sum of money is after income tax and national

insurance have been deducted from earnings and after council tax, rent, mortgage and water charges have been paid. It is, therefore, what a household has available to spend on everything else it needs.

4   Defined here as £6.50 per hour. £6.50 per hour is roughly two-thirds of the Great Britain median hourly earnings and is commonly used as a threshold when analysing low pay.

5   For example, Cabinet Office, Prime Minister's Strategy Unit, *Improving the Life Chances of Disabled People*, 2005 (a joint report with the Department for Work and Pensions, Department of Health, Department for Education and Skills and Office of the Deputy Prime Minister); Office of the Deputy Prime Minister, *Mental Health and Social Exclusion*, 2003; *Attitudes Towards, and Experiences of, Disability in Britain*, DWP Research Report 173, 2002

6   Department for Work and Pensions, *Five Year Strategy: opportunity and security throughout life*, The Stationery Office, 2005, p42

Two
Children with disabled parents
Hugh Stickland and Richard Olsen

Introduction

The strong association between child poverty and parental worklessness is well documented. Roughly half of all children in poverty live in a household where no adult is working. At the same time, it is well acknowledged that worklessness is closely associated with disability and poor health. Compared with Britain's overall employment rate of around 75 per cent,[1] the employment rate for disabled people and those with health conditions is roughly 46 per cent[2] (using the Disability Discrimination Act definition of disability).[3] It is extraordinary, therefore, given the strength of association between disability, worklessness and child poverty, that the place of disabled parents in debates about child poverty, and in strategies and policies designed to challenge it, has been so weak. This is despite the fact that there are around 1.7 million disabled parents[4] in the UK today, and around 2.2 million children[5] in their care. With 17 per cent of children having at least one disabled parent, it is impossible to ignore the sheer scale of this group of families. Statistics estimate that nearly 700,000 children of disabled parents are living in poverty before housing costs.[6]

This chapter considers poverty among children who have a disabled parent and uses data from a variety of sources to compare the effects on child poverty of parental disability, parental worklessness and family composition. Both the composition of those in child poverty, as well as the risk of children in particular sets of circumstances living in poverty are examined. The chapter concludes by arguing that any attempt to reduce child poverty should address poverty among disabled parents.

Policy context

The Government recognises that many disabled people currently receiving incapacity-related benefits would like to work. Not all of them, however, are actually able to work, or can find jobs that suit their particular needs. The Department for Work and Pensions' (DWP) *Five Year Strategy* lays out the Government's plans for helping disabled people move into, and stay in, work. At the same time, the Government has a public service agreement (PSA) target to halve child poverty by 2010, on the way to eradicating it by 2020. In addition, the DWP is committed to a number of other PSA targets, which underpin the above goal. These include commitments to:

- reduce the proportion of children living in workless households by 5 per cent between spring 2005 and spring 2008;
- significantly reduce the difference between disabled people's employment rate and the overall employment rate, taking account of the economic cycle, in the three years to March 2008.

As this chapter will show, disabled parents are important to achieving all these goals. However, while the Government has made specific provision for disabled people, and specific provision for parents, there are no goals, targets, interventions or programmes specifically tailored for disabled parents. Indeed, the way in which (single) parents as one distinct group, and disabled people as another, have been separated in the roll-out of the New Deal is indicative of the way in which parenting and disability have always been constructed as wholly different welfare categories by central government.

Parenting, disability and worklessness

Figure 2.1 shows how the populations of parents, disabled people and workless people in the UK overlap.

The diagram shows that there are approximately 1.7 million disabled parents. This is from a population of 14.1 million parents and a population of 5.6 million disabled people. Thus, around 12 per cent of all parents are disabled parents, and around 30 per cent of all disabled peo-

Figure 2.1

Disability, worklessness and parenthood

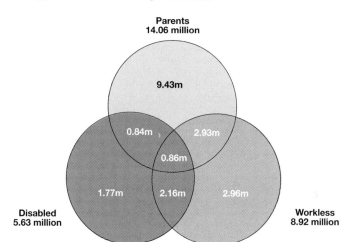

Source: *Labour Force Survey*, National Statistics/Palgrave Macmillan, 2004
www.statistics.gov.uk/STATBASE/Source.asp?vink=358&More=Y

ple also have children and are thus disabled parents. These figures are strikingly similar to figures for the US. In a 1997 survey, disabled parents were found to represent 11 per cent of the 57.9 million parents in the US.[7] The diagram also shows the workless population in Britain. Of the 8.9 million workless people, around one-third (just over three million) are disabled. Around 3.8 million (42 per cent) are parents.

Having already highlighted the link between paid employment and poverty, it is worth reviewing the employment rates of disabled parents and comparing them with other groups, such as non-disabled parents. Employment rates for the key groups are presented in Figure 2.2.

The overall UK employment rate stands at 74.7 per cent. This compares with the employment rate for disabled people of 46.3 per cent. Disabled parents have an employment rate of 49.3 per cent, which compares favourably with that of disabled people as a whole. This possibly reflects the fact that disabled people who are also parents are less likely to be among those disabled people with the most severe impairments who, in turn, are most likely to be out of paid work. However, employment

Figure 2.2

Employment rates of key groups

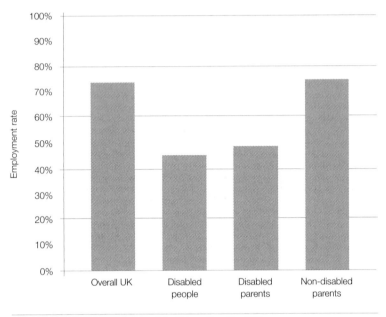

Source: *Labour Force Survey*, National Statistics/Palgrave Macmillan, 2004

rates for disabled parents are some way behind those of non-disabled parents.

It is helpful, however, to consider disabled parents in terms of the households of which they are a part. The 1.7 million disabled parents live in approximately 1.1 million households. This means that, as one would expect, some disabled parents are married to (or cohabiting with) each other. Figure 2.3 shows employment rates by household. For a household to be considered employed, at least one adult in the household must be in paid employment. Similarly, for it to be disabled, at least one adult in the household must be disabled according to the Disability Discrimination Act definition.

Couples with children where neither are disabled have a household employment rate of over 97 per cent. This drops to 78 per cent when at least one of the couple is disabled. Similarly, for non-disabled lone parents the employment rate of almost 60 per cent is significantly higher than for disabled lone parents at 40 per cent. Clearly, then, disability and lone par-

Figure 2.3
Household employment rates

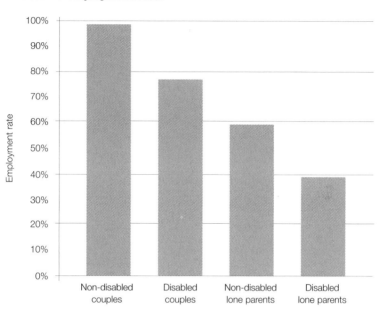

Source: *Labour Force Survey*, National Statistics/Palgrave Macmillan, 2004

enthood have significant effects on the likelihood of households having any economically active adult in them.

Disabled parents and child poverty

There are 12.5 million children in Britain today, of which 2.6 million (before housing costs – BHC) and 3.5 million (after housing costs – AHC) are classed as being in poverty. Such figures are based on official definitions of poverty defined by having an income less than 60 per cent of the contemporary equivalised[8] median. Of the 12.5 million children, 2.1 million (17 per cent) have disabled parents. Table 2.1 shows the composition of the group of children in poverty, together with the risk[9] of being in poverty for children with disabled parents.

Table 2.1
Disabled parents and child poverty

	Before housing costs	After housing costs
Number of children in poverty	2,600,000	3,500,000
Number of children in poverty who have a disabled parent	700,000	800,000
% of all children in poverty living with disabled parents	25%	23%
Total number of children in Britain	12,500,000	12,500,000
Total number of children with disabled parents	2,100,000	2,100,000
Risk of child poverty for all children with disabled parents	30%	38%
Total number of children without disabled parents	10,400,000	10,400,000
Risk of child poverty for all children with non-disabled parents	19%	26%

Source: Department for Work and Pensions, *Households Below Average Income 1994/05-2003/04*,
Corporate Document Services, 2005

There is some debate about whether before or after housing costs should carry more weight when discussing poverty, which is also applicable to disabled parents. One could argue that disabled people might experience higher housing costs, because of specific needs or alterations. However, while Table 2.1 shows that the risk of poverty increases for children with disabled parents when switching between BHC and AHC, this is mirrored by a similar increase for children of non-disabled parents. When comparing disabled and non-disabled parents, the two measures will give similar results and, therefore, the following concentrates on the BHC measure. Measures for the 2010/11 target will also include material deprivation, and analysis will be needed to see whether these pick out any further effects that disability may have.

The composition of overall child poverty on both BHC and AHC measures shows that roughly one-quarter of children in poverty have disabled parents, and three-quarters have non-disabled parents. However, when considering the risk of child poverty, the importance of disabled parents becomes more apparent. On the BHC measure, 700,000 of the 2.1 million children with disabled parents are in poverty. This means the risk of poverty for children with a disabled parent is 30 per cent. This increases to 38 per cent when using the AHC measure. In comparison, the risk of poverty for children with non-disabled parents is 19 per cent BHC and 26 per cent AHC. Again, these figures demonstrate that the risk of children experiencing poverty is significantly increased when they have at least one disabled parent. However, a cautionary note is required here: the risk of all children experiencing poverty has diminished in recent years, and the risk of the children of disabled parents experiencing poverty has also reduced. The children of disabled parents are still much more likely to experience poverty, but this group has benefited from reductions in overall child poverty.

Poverty by family type

The Government's measure of child poverty is those children who live in households whose income is 60 per cent or less of the median income. This section uses this measure to consider disabled parents and poverty in more detail.

Table 2.2

Composition and risk of child poverty by family type (BHC)

Adult disability by family type and economic status		Children in poverty	
		Composition	**Risk**
Workless lone parent	Disabled adults	7%	49%
	No disabled adults	22%	51%
Workless couple	Disabled adults	9%	57%
	No disabled adults	8%	73%
Working lone parent	Disabled adults	2%	20%
	No disabled adults	7%	14%
Working couple	Disabled adults	9%	17%
	No disabled adults	36%	12%

Source: Department for Work and Pensions, *Households Below Average Income 1994/05-2003/04*, Corporate Document Services, 2005

There is a wealth of data in Table 2.2, which we can break down by the three variables given (working/workless, couple/lone parent and disabled/non-disabled). There is also information on the composition of the 2.6 million children in poverty broken down by these groups, and information on the risk of poverty for children in each of these groups. First, looking at composition, poverty can be broken down by the three main groups. Forty-six per cent of children in poverty live in workless households, whereas 54 per cent live in working households. Thirty-eight per cent of children in poverty live in lone-parent households, whereas 62 per cent live in couple households. Twenty-seven per cent of children in poverty have at least one disabled parent, whereas 73 per cent do not have a disabled parent.

Looking at workless lone-parent households, the composition shows that the majority of children in poverty have a non-disabled lone parent. We know that roughly 20 per cent of workless lone parents are disabled, which is consistent with the figures in the table above. The risk of poverty for children in workless lone-parent households is high, but almost equal between disabled and non-disabled lone parents (49 per cent and 51 per cent respectively). This small difference may be due to some disabled lone parents qualifying for incapacity-related benefits, which may boost their out-of-work income above that of non-disabled lone parents receiving income support.

The risk of child poverty decreases substantially when a lone parent moves into work and this is reflected by the fact that there are fewer children in poverty in working lone-parent households as compared with workless lone-parent households. Wages and working tax credit (WTC) raise income levels in lone-parent households, resulting in the risk of poverty falling to 14 per cent for children in non-disabled lone-parent households, and 20 per cent for children in disabled lone-parent households. The effects of disability on employment and poverty will be discussed later, when considering working couples.

Sixty-two per cent of children living in poverty live in couple households. Perhaps unexpectedly, the majority of these (45 per cent) live in households where at least one of the adults is working. The remaining 17 per cent live in workless households.

Of those children living in poverty who live in a workless couple household, just over half have at least one disabled parent. However, we know that of all workless couple households with children, two-thirds have at least one disabled parent (see Figure 2.4 below).

These figures imply that there is a greater risk for children in workless couple households without disabled parents to be in poverty compared with children in workless couple households with at least one disabled parent. This is confirmed in the risk figures, with 73 per cent of children in non-disabled workless couple households at risk of poverty, compared with 57 per cent where there is at least one disabled parent (see Table 2.2).

Figure 2.4
Workless households and disabled parents[10]

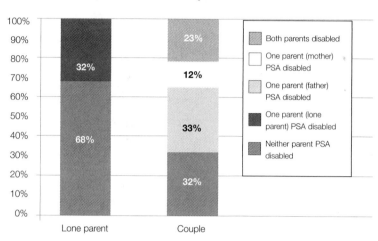

Source: *Labour Force Survey*, National Statistics/Palgrave Macmillan, 2003

Workless couple households where neither parent is disabled are most likely to be claiming jobseeker's allowance (JSA). Workless couple households with at least one disabled parent are likely to be in receipt of an incapacity-related benefit. JSA is designed to be a short-term benefit for those looking for and gaining employment. Couples with children who are dependent on JSA as their main source of income will almost certainly find themselves in poverty. This explains why the risk of poverty for this group is extremely high (with 73 per cent of children in these households in poverty). However, the majority of non-disabled workless couples remain on benefit and are out of work for a short period of time – for example, six months or less (see Table 2.3).

Children in poverty in workless couple families where at least one parent is disabled are most likely to be in households dependent on incapacity-related benefits. While these benefits are more generous than JSA (typically long-term incapacity benefit (IB) is paid at £78.50 a week, with increases for adult and child dependants, compared with £57.45 a week for JSA (2006/07 rates)), reliance on benefit still means that 57 per cent of children in workless couple households with at least one disabled parent are in poverty. The longer-term nature of these benefits also means that

Table 2.3

Duration of benefit receipt for couples with children by benefit type

	Unemployment benefit	Incapacity-related benefit	Others	Total
Under 6 months	18%	5%	2%	25%
6 months to 1 year	6%	4%	1%	11%
1 year to 2 years	5%	7%	1%	13%
2 years plus	3%	44%	4%	51%
Total	32%	60%	8%	

Source: Department for Work and Pensions, *Client Group Analysis Statistics*, National Statistics, 2004

the children may well experience longer, and in some cases much longer, spells of being poor (see Table 2.3).

It should be noted that for both disabled and non-disabled parents who are out of work, additional benefits and payments are available, such as housing benefit, council tax benefit and child tax credit (CTC). Those families who claim these are less likely to be in, or at risk of, poverty.

So, the risk of poverty is lower for children living in workless couple households where there are disabled parents, than where the parents are non-disabled. This is most likely due to differences in the levels at which the different benefits are paid. However, children whose parents are dependent on JSA are likely to be on benefit for shorter durations before moving into employment and, therefore, often out of poverty. In some senses, there will always be couples with children moving in and out of employment, and thus children who are temporarily in poverty because of the low level of financial assistance available via JSA. In contrast, children in a workless couple household with disabled parents are likely to be dependent on benefit for much longer periods, and some parents may never move into work. Thus, although the risk of poverty for this group is lower, the likelihood of being in, or near, poverty lasts for much longer.

Table 2.2 shows that 45 per cent of children in the UK living in poverty live in couple households where at least one adult is working. The majority of these households will have one adult working either at a low wage rate (at or around minimum wage levels) or a limited number of hours, or both. This composition is high because the majority of children in Britain live in working couple households.

The risk of poverty falls dramatically for couples who move from worklessness to employment – from 73 per cent to 12 per cent for non-disabled couples, and from 57 per cent to 17 per cent for disabled couples. However, the risk of poverty is now significantly higher for children with disabled parents than for children with non-disabled parents. This is also true for the children of disabled working lone parents (20 per cent) compared with those of non-disabled working lone parents (14 per cent).

This means that while having a disabled parent in a workless household can insulate children from the likelihood of experiencing poverty (compared with children of non-disabled parents in workless households), having a disabled parent in a household where at least one parent works makes poverty more likely (again compared with being in a non-disabled working household). One reason for this may be the amount and/or type of work open to disabled parents. The likelihood is that disabled parents are more likely to find low-paid and/or part-time work compared with non-disabled parents. This is supported by evidence gathered by the Disability Rights Commission which showed that one-third of disabled people aged 18 to 24 expect to earn less that their non-disabled peers by the age of 30.[11] Furthermore, the employment opportunities of the non-disabled partner of a disabled parent may be affected, particularly if employment has to be combined not only with arranging childcare (as for all families), but also with looking after the disabled parent. These effects on parent and partner employment give non-disabled parents a greater chance of leaving poverty when entering work than disabled parents.

Children whose parents receive wages and tax credits are much less likely to be in poverty than children whose parents receive out-of-work benefits. Take-up of WTC and CTC is relatively high among those families who are eligible. Roughly 4.5 million in-work families are in receipt of WTC and/or CTC. However, the disabled elements of WTC have not been as popular with those who are eligible; just 42,000 in-work families with children are in receipt of the disabled element of WTC. This means that disabled parents moving into work who do not take up the appropriate tax credits may be up to £2,040 per year worse off than if they did.[12]

Additional costs

Of course, in addition to the evidence provided by the data so far, it is important to acknowledge the additional costs involved in being a disabled parent. These may serve further to increase the likelihood of the children of disabled parents experiencing poverty in a way not captured by the discussion so far.

It is likely that some disabled people face higher costs in order to maintain a given standard of living that non-disabled people do not face. These higher costs may include extra fuel costs, mobility costs or additional personal care costs which are associated with having a disability but do not yield a higher standard of living compared with the case where there is no disability. Such extra costs will, in some instances, be at least partly mitigated for through additional benefit payments. However, since the additional benefit payments are considered as income and are not discounted for the extra costs of disability, the extent of poverty among the disabled population may be underestimated.[13]

Disabled parents may face additional expenditure in relation to their parenting role. This includes the cost of buying specialised equipment, the cost of having to buy more expensive models of ordinary equipment and/or the cost of adapting existing equipment. This additional cost could relate to household appliances such as baby bottle sterilisers, cots, stair gates and so on, and to the broader paraphernalia of parenting including pushchairs, safety reins, car seats and so on. As an example, a disabled parent may need to rely on several stair gates to prevent access to parts of the house for a young child when other parents would rely on one stair gate and their mobility to ensure safety.

In addition, disabled parents may need to rely on more expensive convenience and/or takeaway food. This may be because their impairments, or lack of support, make preparation of fresh food more difficult. It may also be because they are less easily able to travel between different retailers in order to take advantage of special offers or economies of scale. When they do travel further distances to shop, it is also more likely to involve costly taxi journeys.

Disabled parents may also face additional household running costs. For instance, an inaccessible garden may make it less easy for them to hang out washing in good weather, requiring extra reliance on tumble dryers. Similarly, they may also face extra telephone costs, given problems in accessing leisure facilities with their children and the need for often lengthy calls in making travel arrangements or arranging trips.

In summary, then, while the evidence linking parental disability and child poverty is very robust, it would be more so if we were able fully to unpack the additional cost of being a disabled parent. The kinds of additional costs faced by disabled parents will vary depending on circumstances. It is clear, however, that there is at least the potential for additional costs not faced by non-disabled parents and, moreover, not faced by disabled people who are not parents.

Conclusions

The parenting role of disabled adults has attracted increasing attention from policy makers and academics over the last decade or so. This is evident in growing research literature.[14] It is also evident in growing central government concern with disabled parents. This includes the Social Services Inspectorate inspections of services for disabled parents resulting in *A Jigsaw of Services*[15] and in the inclusion of disabled parents in *Fair Access to Care Services* guidance. This is coupled with greater activity in local authorities, in particular, to recognise this group and to address some of the barriers they face in fulfilling their parenting role. However, the place of parental disability as a key predictor of child poverty has hitherto received little attention.

The data presented in this chapter leads to certain conclusions regarding the impact of parental disability on child poverty. First, children with disabled parents face a significantly higher risk of living in poverty when compared with the children of non-disabled parents. This is true for households with couples and with lone parents. The primary reason for this is the fact that work plays such a significant role in keeping families out of poverty, and that disabled parents are much less likely to be in paid work.

Second, the children of disabled parents in workless families are somewhat less likely to be living in poverty than children in workless families without disabled parents. The most likely explanation is the higher levels at which IB is paid compared with JSA. However, although the benefits system is more generous to disabled parents than non-disabled parents, spells of poverty are likely to be much longer for children with disabled parents, given that reliance on IB is generally much more long term than are spells of unemployment for non-disabled parents. The families of disabled parents who are not able to work should receive an income above the poverty line after considering additional costs of parenting and disability, thus ensuring 'security for those who can't work'.

Third, when their parents move into work, the risk of poverty is greater for children with disabled parents than those with non-disabled parents. The most likely cause is the relatively low-paid, part-time and insecure work that disabled people are more likely to take. This discrimination in employment opportunities carries over to non-disabled partners who are more likely to find themselves juggling employment with both parenting and caring responsibilities, jeopardising the levels of income they can attract.

Although disabled parents are key to achieving a number of policy goals and targets, they often fall between the gaps of provision for disabled people and provision for parents. For central government initiatives to tackle child poverty to be successful, the poverty experienced by disabled parents has to receive greater attention. This could be done in a number of ways, including reviewing the way in which disability-related benefits take into account the additional costs of being a disabled parent, and taking measures to ensure that employment opportunities are fully open to disabled people.

Notes

1 *Labour Force Survey*, National Statistics/Palgrave Macmillan, 2004 – 74.7 per cent

2 See note 1 – 46.3 per cent

3 A person has a disability if he has a physical or mental impairment which has a substantial and long-term adverse effect on his ability to carry out normal day-to-day activities.

4 See note 1

5 Department for Work and Pensions, *Households Below Average Income 1994/95-2003/04*, Corporate Document Services, 2005

6 See note 5

7 L Toms-Barker and V Maralani, *Challenges and Strategies of Disabled Parents: findings from a national survey of parents with disabilities*, Through the Looking Glass, 1977

8 Equivalised income is income that has undergone a process by which it is adjusted to account for variations in household size and composition. Income is divided by scales that vary according to the number of adults, and the number and age of dependants in the household.

9 Risk is the chance of individuals in a group falling below a given threshold. It is calculated as the number in the group below the given threshold divided by the total number in the group.

10 PSA definition of disabled, which refers to both Disability Discrimination Act-disabled and those with a work-limiting disability.

11 L Sayce, *Disability Rights and Disabled Parents*, Disability Rights Commission, 2004, available at www.drc-gb.org/publicationsandreports/campaigndetails.asp?section=emp&id=446

12 Inland Revenue, *Child and Working Tax Credits Quarterly Statistics*, National Statistics, December 2004

13 This is a complex area and readers are encouraged to refer to additional work, such as G Preston, *Family Values: disabled parents, extra costs and the benefit system*, Disability Alliance, 2005

14 R Olsen and H Clarke, *Parenting and Disability: disabled parents' experiences of raising children*, The Policy Press, 2003; R Olsen and H Tyers, *Think Parent! Supporting disabled adults as parents*, National Family and Parenting Institute/ Joseph Rowntree Foundation, 2004; R Olsen and M Wates, *Disabled Parents: examining research assumptions*, Research Review 6, Research in Practice, 2003; M Wates, *Disabled Parents: dispelling the myths*, National Childbirth Trust/Radcliffe Medical Press, 1997; M Wates, *Supporting Disabled Adults in their Parenting Role*, Joseph Rowntree Foundation, 2002

15 S Goodinge, *A Jigsaw of Services: inspection of services to support disabled adults in their parenting role*, Social Services Inspectorate, 2000

Three

Changing weights and measures: disability and child poverty

Tania Burchardt

This chapter considers how poverty affects children with disabled parents, and disabled children relative to children not affected by disability. It considers why there are high levels of poverty among children affected by disability, questions whether *Households Below Average Income* (HBAI) data allows accurate comparisons to be made between different household types – particularly between households affected and unaffected by disability – and considers whether the Department for Work and Pensions' (DWP) new measure of material deprivation will resolve current shortcomings in statistical data on poverty.

Poverty among children affected by disability

Since 1999/00, the HBAI series has published breakdowns of poverty rates by disability status. Interpretation of these depends on whether one concentrates on *levels* of poverty or on *rates of change.* In terms of levels, it remains the case that children living in households with one or more disabled adults are significantly more likely to be living on a low income than children in households with no disabled adult (38 per cent compared with 26 per cent). Children who are themselves disabled, or who have a disabled sibling, are also at greater risk of poverty (31 per cent compared with 27 per cent of those in households with no disabled children). Finally, children living in households containing both a disabled child and a disabled adult, although they make up only 4 per cent of all children, are at high risk of poverty. At the beginning of the period, half were living under the poverty line (defined here as 60 per cent of median income after housing costs), falling to 36 per cent in the most recent figures. There is clearly much more to be done, both in terms of closing the gap between children affected by disability and the rest, and in terms of the overall levels of poverty among all groups of children.

Table 3.1:
Trends in child poverty rates, by household composition

			Children in households			
Year	All children	No disabled adult	One or more disabled adults	No disabled child	One or more disabled children	Disabled adult and disabled child
1999/00[1]	32	29	45	31	40	50
2000/01	30	28	43	30	36	39[2]
2001/02	30	27	43	29	35	46
2002/03	28	26	39	28	31	40
2003/04	28	26	38	27	31	36
Composition of child population (%)	*100*	*83*	*17*	*90*	*10*	*4*

Source: Department for Work and Pensions, *Households Below Average Income1994/95 – 2003/04*, Corporate Document Services, 2005 and previous editions

[1] Figures exclude the self-employed.

[2] This figure is out of line with the trend and may reflect sampling or clerical error in the series.

On the other hand, looking at the rates of change in poverty over this five-year period, the picture is more encouraging. Rates of poverty have fallen faster for groups of children affected by disability than for other children, with the result that the gaps between them have narrowed. Overall rates of poverty for children fell by 12.5 per cent, but for children in a household with a disabled adult the decline was 15.6 per cent, for disabled children (or with a disabled sibling) it was 22.5 per cent, and for children with both a disabled adult and a disabled child in the household it was 28 per cent. Of course, these decreases were from a higher initial level, so larger changes are, arguably, easier to achieve, but it is nevertheless to be welcomed that there has been both a convergence in the rates of poverty among children affected by disability and the rest, and an overall fall.

There is nothing inevitable about these changes. Indeed, if one turns to the figures for adults of working age (not shown in Table 3.1), poverty rates among disabled adults and those living with a disabled adult have fallen only very slightly to 28 per cent, while the rate for adults unaffected by disability has risen slightly to 17 per cent. The result is a slight narrowing in poverty rates between the two groups, but for the wrong reason – by increasing poverty among the previously less at-risk group.

Equivalisation and the extra costs of disability

The figures from the HBAI series are the mainstay of monitoring child poverty. However, there are concerns about whether they allow accurate comparisons to be made between different household types, and particularly between households affected and unaffected by disability.

The HBAI series adjusts incomes for differences in household size and composition – a process known as equivalisation. The idea is to take account of the fact that a larger household is likely to have a lower standard of living than a smaller household with the same income. At present, the adjustments are made according to the McClements scale, but the next release of HBAI data in 2007 will use alternative scales. These make international comparisons easier and give greater weight to the costs of babies (which the McClements scale is widely thought to undercount) and will lead to an increase in the estimated rates of poverty of about one percentage point.[1]

It is difficult to predict how the change in equivalisation will affect comparisons between the poverty rates of disabled and non-disabled children. Probably more significant for that comparison is the fact that neither the old nor the new scales take account of the extra costs of living incurred by families with a disabled adult or child. Estimates of the extra costs of disability have varied widely. The most recent research presented estimates based on a budget standards approach, ranging from £389 per week for someone with 'low-medium needs' to £1,513 for someone with high-medium mobility needs and personal assistance.[2] Previous estimates using alternative methods ranged from 14 per cent of income for someone with low severity impairments, to 78 per cent for someone with high severity (figures for single non-pensioners).[3]

There have been fewer attempts to quantify the extra costs of disabled children, but in-depth qualitative work indicates that they are considerable.[4] Depending on the nature of the child's impairment, they may range from additional childcare costs (because of the lack of availability of suitable places), through to the cost of replacing furniture and items of equipment more frequently, to costs of therapies not available on the NHS but which parents feel are very valuable to their child.

Some benefits are available to help towards the extra costs of disability, in particular, disability living allowance (DLA). This is included in the calculation of income in the HBAI series, but the extra costs of living that it is designed to meet are not. Thus, disabled people (and others in households containing a disabled person) appear to be better off in the HBAI figures than they really are, at least in terms of the standard of living they can hope to obtain on the income they receive.

The principle of equivalisation for disability is the same as that for differences in household size and composition, yet, so far, the DWP has resisted incorporating any adjustment for disability into the main estimates. An appendix to HBAI regularly reports the sensitivity of overall poverty rates to including an additional factor of 0.10 for each disabled adult or child to the household equivalisation factor, but this figure is, as the publication itself states, arbitrary, and according to many of the studies described above, too low. Moreover, no breakdown of the results of the sensitivity analysis by disability status is provided.

Low income and deprivation

Current measures of child poverty leave a great deal to be desired when it comes to comparisons between families affected by disability and others. Perhaps the new measure of child poverty, due to be produced by the Spending Review 2007, will help. After consultation with CPAG among others, the DWP determined that the pledge to end child poverty would be measured against progress on three scales.[5]

- **Absolute income.** The poverty threshold fixed at 1998/99 levels and uprated only in line with inflation. This means that the income of a family on the poverty threshold should buy the same basket of goods in 2005/06 as in 1998/99, but it does not take into account any changes in expectations of what a family needs.
- **Relative income.** The poverty threshold set relative to contemporary median income. This indicates whether children are keeping pace with the general rise in standards of living.

- **Material deprivation.** Families who lack certain goods and services and have an income below 70 per cent of median income.

Material deprivation is the most innovative component of the new DWP measure. The precise list of goods and services is yet to be determined, but will be drawn from those listed in Table 3.2. Survey respondents who say they would like to have the item in question but cannot afford it will be classified as lacking that item. The number of items a family must lack in order to count as deprived has also yet to be determined.

Table 3.2

Items from which an index of material deprivation will be drawn

Adult deprivation	Child deprivation
Keep your home in a decent state of repair	Enough bedrooms for every child over 10 of different sex to have her/his own bedroom
Keep your home adequately warm	Celebrations on special occasions, such as birthdays, Christmas or other religious festivals
Replace any worn-out furniture	Play group/nursery/toddler group at least once a week for children of pre-school age
Replace or repair broken electrical goods, such as refrigerator or washing machine	Going on a school trip at least once a term for school-aged children
Two pairs of all-weather shoes	Leisure equipment (for example, sports equipment or a bicycle)
Holiday away from home for one week per year, not staying with relatives	Holiday away from home at least one week per year with her/his family
Have friends and family for a drink or meal at least once a month	Friends round for tea or a snack once a fortnight
Hobby or leisure activity	Hobby or leisure activity
Small amount of money to spend each week on yourself, not on your family	Swimming at least once a month
Regular savings (of £10 a month) for rainy days or retirement	
Insurance of contents of dwelling	

Source: Department for Work and Pensions, *Measuring Child Poverty*, 2003

The motivation for using an index of deprivation is two-fold. Firstly, it is thought that deprivation has more intuitive meaning to the general public than poverty expressed as a percentage of mean or median income. This may be so in principle, although by the time one has explained a family who is counted as deprived must say that they lack a certain number of a list of items which they want but cannot afford and that their income is less than 70 per cent of median income, any intuitive appeal may have been lost. The second reason for adopting a deprivation measure is that the DWP, and some of the experts it consulted, was concerned about inaccuracy in the measurement of low incomes. Some people on a low income appear to have relatively high standards of living. Questions like those in Table 3.2 attempt to measure standards of living directly. However, this approach raises a number of its own difficulties. Firstly, respondents must say that they want the item in question. But this does not allow for the possibility that people's expectations are conditioned by their circumstances.

Secondly, respondents who say they do want an item (for example, to take their child swimming) are then asked whether the reason they do not is because they cannot afford it. There are many barriers to participation other than affordability, particularly for disabled people, which will not be picked up by this measure of deprivation. The swimming pool may be inaccessible or unsafe, or there may be no transport available to get there. Families with disabled children (or parents) who are prevented from participating for these reasons will not be classified as deprived by the DWP formula.

Thirdly, combining the deprivation measure with an income threshold, as the DWP intends, means that those who have a low standard of living, despite having a slightly higher income, will not be classified as deprived. This again is problematic for comparisons between disabled and non-disabled children and families. A family in receipt of extra-costs benefits like DLA may have an income above the poverty threshold (in this case, 70 per cent of median income) but, nevertheless, be unable to afford or access a number of the items listed because of the extra costs they incur. Such a family will be excluded from the deprivation figures by the income cut-off.

Deprivation measures have the potential to improve comparisons between families who are and who are not affected by disability because they *can* focus on the extent to which families are able to access goods, services, and activities, which gets to the heart of the idea of social inclusion. Unfortunately, the particular form of deprivation indicator on which the DWP has settled does not help to meet this objective, because it focuses on affordability rather than accessibility, and because it re-introduces an income threshold without making any allowance for extra costs.

Aspirations and employment of disabled young people

One might anticipate that disabled children growing up with all the frustrations of inaccessible transport and venues, unhelpful social attitudes and so on, combined with the constraints imposed by living in a family on a low income, would look ahead to adult life with little enthusiasm and with a limited range of ideas about the roles they could play. But recent research funded by the Joseph Rowntree Foundation has found that today's disabled teenagers have high aspirations for their further education and later employment.[6]

In one survey, three-fifths of disabled young people wanted to stay on in education at age 16, the same proportion as non-disabled young people. Between one in three and one in four of each group aspired to a professional occupation, and both groups felt that getting a good job would be an important component of adult life. The average weekly pay disabled and non-disabled teenagers expected to be able to get from a full-time job was the same.

These results are particularly encouraging because previous research on disabled teenagers in the 1960s had found disabled young people's aspirations were significantly lower than their non-disabled counterparts.[7] So it seems the 'aspiration gap' between disabled and non-disabled young people has narrowed over time. One can speculate that this might be the result of greater integration in education, and the increased prominence of the disability rights movement.

Unfortunately, when we turn to the experience of these same young people as they move into adulthood, the picture is less rosy. By age 18/19, disabled young people are nearly three times as likely to be unemployed or 'doing something else' as their non-disabled counterparts, widening to nearly four times as likely by age 26. Those who had been able to find work were earning 11 per cent less than their non-disabled counterparts, even after taking into account differences in educational qualifications.

Despite their high aspirations, it seems as if the employment opportunities are not available for these disabled people in early adulthood. Many will be surviving on a low income, possibly continuing to live with parents, and claiming incapacity benefit (IB). Any help with turning their aspirations for fulfilling employment into a reality by the Government is, of course, to be welcomed.

Unfortunately, the aspects of the proposed reforms which have emerged so far seem unlikely to meet this objective. Two features are clear. Firstly, some claimants will be required to undertake some form of job-seeking/preparation activities as a condition of receiving their benefit. Secondly, the emphasis will continue to be on the claimant adapting her/himself to the world of work, rather than the other way round. These young people do not need to be compelled to look for work; they have stated their desire to work and often formulated quite detailed plans about how they want to achieve their aim. Neither will nor commitment are lacking, but the substantive opportunities for good quality jobs are. Rather than preaching to the already-converted claimants, IB personal advisers might spend their time more productively ensuring that employers are well informed about their duties under the Disability Discrimination Act, and aware of the financial help available to them to make any necessary adjustments to employ a disabled person through the Access to Work scheme.

Conclusion

The high profile of policies on child poverty and on disability has not, as yet, resulted in a significant degree of 'joining up' between the two. There have been improvements – disabled young people today are more positive about their future lives than their counterparts in earlier generations, and the recent narrowing of the gaps in poverty rates between disabled and non-disabled children, and between children of disabled and non-disabled parents, is certainly to be welcomed. But both the measurement of child poverty (and its relationship to disability) and the overall shape of proposed benefit reforms continue to be unhelpful. Until the statistics reflect the extra costs of disability, meaningful conclusions about relative living standards across different families are difficult to draw. And until welfare-to-work policies acknowledge that, for young people at least, the problem lies not with their motivation but with the lack of substantive opportunities available to them, the aspirations of disabled young people will remain frustrated.

Notes

1 Department for Work and Pensions, *Households Below Average Income Statistics: adoption of new equivalence scales*, HBAI team First Release, 2005
2 N Smith, S Middleton, K Ashton-Brooks, L Cox and B Dobson with L Reith, *Disabled People's Costs of Living: 'more than you would think'*, The Policy Press for Joseph Rowntree Foundation, 2004

3 A Zaidi and T Burchardt, 'Comparing Incomes When Needs Differ: equivalising for the extra costs of disability in the UK', *Review of Income and Wealth*, 51(1), 2005 pp89-114

4 G Preston, *Helter Skelter: families, disabled children and the benefit system*, CASEpaper 92, Centre for Analysis of Social Exclusion, London School of Economics, 2005

5 Department for Work and Pensions, *Measuring Child Poverty*, 2003

6 T Burchardt, *The Education and Employment of Disabled Young People: frustrated ambition*, The Policy Press, 2005

7 A Walker, *Unqualified and Underemployed: handicapped young people and the labour market*, Macmillan, 1982

Four
Living with disability: a message from disabled parents

Gabrielle Preston

The recently published Green Paper on welfare reform outlines the Government's strategy to move one million disabled people off incapacity benefits within a decade and increase significantly the number of disabled people in paid employment.[1] There are currently just over two million disabled parents in the UK. Around half of these (one million) are also workless, accounting for one in three out-of-work disabled adults.[2] Addressing the particular barriers disabled parents face to employment is crucial if the Government is to meet this ambitious target.

This chapter considers welfare reform from the perspective of disabled adults with parenting responsibilities. The first section provides a brief overview of government policy on disabled parents and child poverty. The second part draws directly on the personal experiences and viewpoints of a small number of disabled parents interviewed for this work. It outlines the impact that disability has on parents' and children's lives; records parents' attitudes to, and experiences of, paid employment; questions the accessibility and adequacy of disability benefits, including incapacity benefit (IB); and considers the availability and appropriateness of services. It examines whether the proposals outlined in the Green Paper are likely to assist more disabled parents into work, and whether they will help or hinder the Government's policy on reducing child poverty. It concludes with a number of key messages from disabled parents for the Government.

Parents in this study experienced a range of disabilities, including physical disabilities, learning disabilities and mental health problems. A number of parents expressed discomfort with the term 'disabled', which possibly reflects a tendency to view the term as a medical rather than a social condition. As one parent observed, 'I know I am disabled, but I don't term myself disabled unless somebody makes me disabled...' A distinction should be drawn between impairments and health conditions, and 'disability' (which arises out of society's failure to respond to the needs of people with impairments). Many disabled parents feel positive about their qualifications, experiences and skills, and emphasise that they are disabled by discrimination rather than their physical or mental impairment. In this chapter, for reasons of clarity, all participating parents are referred to as 'disabled parents'.

Introduction

The Government accepts that children with sick or disabled parents are vulnerable to living in poverty, that disabled parents are particularly disadvantaged in the labour market, and that children with disabled parents face a disproportionate risk of living in poverty.[3] The *Child Poverty Review*, published as part of Spending Review 2004, reports that:

> Parenting support is especially important for poor parents in vulnerable groups such as disabled parents, who face a particular risk of being in poverty. Over two million children live in families with one or more disabled adults. These children have an above average risk of living in low-income households.[4]

Improving the Life Chances of Disabled People records that:

> Among workless households with children, the majority have at least one disabled parent: children are more likely to experience poverty if there are disabled adults in the family.[5]

The recently published *Households Below Average Income* data indicates that, after housing costs have been accounted for, 24 per cent of the 3.4 million poor children in Great Britain (around 816,000) lived with one or more disabled adult in 2004/05. The risk of income poverty for this group was 40 per cent (against an average risk for all children of 27 per cent).[6]

The Government believes that 'helping parents into work is the most sustainable way to tackle child poverty and give children better opportunities to succeed in later life.'[7] However, the Department for Work and Pensions (DWP) accepts that accessing employment is particularly difficult for disabled parents. In November 2003, the DWP and the Treasury organised a high-level seminar, which considered the many barriers disabled parents face to the labour market, including low qualifications, poor service provision (for example, childcare and social services for personal assistance), additional disability-related costs and problems with transport.[8] The DWP highlighted the fact that disabled lone parents experience additional problems.[9]

A paper circulated at the seminar concluded that:

> Whilst the Government recognises and has put in place strategies to raise the employment rate of disabled people, reduce the number of children in workless households and reduce child poverty, strategies to help disabled people return to work do not make specific provision for those who are also parents; nor do strategies for lone and couple parents make specific provision for those who are disabled.[10]

The Government accepts that it is difficult to discuss employment strategies for disabled people without considering support services. However, disabled parents are particularly disadvantaged in this respect.

In April 2000 the Social Services Inspectorate published *A Jigsaw of Services: inspection of services to support disabled adults in their parenting role*, which highlighted a lack of flexible services to support disabled people undertake their parenting role. Although a task force was set up by the Joseph Rowntree Foundation with the support of the Department of Health to identify how best to support disabled adults in their parenting role[11] and a recent report published by the Department of Health[12] seeks to resolve these sorts of problems, the disabled parents interviewed reported that their parenting responsibilities are routinely ignored by services and have not been taken into consideration in the Green Paper.

Improving the Life Chances of Disabled People emphasises that 'recognising the particular needs and circumstances of disabled parents will be vital to the achievement of policy objectives of increasing employment rates and tackling child poverty'[13] and yet the Green Paper does not engage with the needs of disabled parents. Clearly, if the Government wishes to succeed in its two very ambitious targets – drawing one million disabled people off incapacity benefits, and halving child poverty by 2010 – policy initiatives must consider the needs of disabled parents.

The case studies

Although the parents who participated in this small study are by no means representative, they illustrate the fact that disabled parents span many groups that are at risk of living in poverty. Parents interviewed include couples, lone parents, parents with disabled children, parents with additional caring responsibilities, parents with larger families and parents from black and minority ethnic groups. Some parents experienced additional disadvantages, such as domestic violence, teenage pregnancy and homelessness. The parents cover a wide age range.

The families

The names of all parents and children have been changed.

Ginny is a disabled parent whose husband is in full-time employment. Although Ginny worked for nearly 25 years, she gave up work when a deteriorating medical condition and parenting two very young children had a negative impact on both her long-term health and the quality of her parenting. She has not returned to paid employment because loss of benefit would need to be offset by full-time employment, which she is no longer physically able to sustain. Ginny is currently organising a peer support group of disabled parents in her local authority area on a voluntary basis.

Louise is a disabled parent whose husband is in full-time employment. Louise has always worked, most recently in a demanding professional capacity for a large government agency. Six months ago Louise developed a secondary impairment, which necessitated a number of adaptations at work. Managing a full-time job without adequate support alongside parenting proved to be too much and Louise was forced to give up her job. She is currently looking for work, but she fears that if she does succeed in getting a job it will be well below her skill levels. Louise has two daughters.

Liz and Bill are both disabled. They live with their 10-year-old daughter, Alexandra. **Liz** previously worked as a carer and was hoping to train as a nurse, but her health problems mean that she is unable to undertake any kind of physical work. She is currently studying IT, which she hopes will enable her to do some voluntary work. **Bill** was a skilled fitter before being made redundant some years ago. After working for a short time as a kitchen porter, he moved onto IB after a major work-related back injury. Bill was unable to maintain the mortgage payments and the family lost their home. Bill cares for Liz, his elderly mother and his daughter. Although high levels of stress have generated additional health problems, Bill is hoping to retrain and to access employment with the help of his disability personal adviser.

Susie is a lone parent with mental health problems. She worked full time for 20 years, during which time she was regularly admitted to psychiatric hospitals. Her relationship broke down after her first hospital admission and Susie was unable to combine working and parenting her two-year-old daughter, Anna, who was looked after by her grandmother. Susie gave up work three years ago after another hospital admission. Her daughter now lives with her. Susie runs a service user group.

Anna, Susie's 17-year-old daughter is studying for her A levels. Anna has lived with her grandmother since she was two and saw her parents – who are separated – at the weekends. Anna moved in with Susie after she gave up full-time employment three years ago.

Rose is severely disabled and is a wheelchair user. She lives with her husband, John, and they have four children. Her son, Steven, has leukaemia and has been in and out of hospital for treatment for two years. John gave up full-time employment two years ago so that he could stay with Steven in hospital and the family now live on benefits.

Amrit is a 23-year-old South East Asian lone parent with mental health problems who has a three-year-old daughter. Although Amrit did well at school, her education was disrupted by mental health and family problems. Although she is keen to complete her academic training, regular hospital admissions and problems with housing have rendered it difficult for her to fulfill her academic potential. Amrit is finding it difficult to balance being a full-time mother with studying and/or working.

Sally is a 22-year-old lone parent with mental health problems. She has a three-year-old daughter. She moved out of her family home when she was 15. Although she started a university degree, she had to give up because of lack of support for her as a parent. Sally would like to complete her studies and access employment in due course, but for the moment she wants to care for her daughter.

Linda is a lone parent who has chronic back problems that necessitated spinal surgery some years ago. She has two grown up children and an 11-year-old daughter. Linda is currently trying to access employment with the support of her personal adviser at the Jobcentre Plus. Although Linda is very keen to work, she fears that her age (44) and lack of qualifications will render this difficult.

Support group for parents with learning disabilities. We visited a small group of parents with learning disabilities. **Maria** and her husband **William** have four children, one of whom is severely disabled and is a wheelchair user. **Teresa** has mild learning disabilities. Her son is at a special school and her grown-up daughter has Asperger's Syndrome. **Denise**, whose partner has severe mental health problems, has three children, one of whom is disabled. We have included some comments from the facilitator of the group, **Gill**.

Employment

Disabled parents are well aware that the onset of ill-health or a disability is not only associated with a drop in income, but can generate social exclusion. Many would like to do paid work in addition to their role as parents caring for children, and recognise that it can bring significant financial and psychological benefits – including a sense of self-worth and social inclusion. Liz reports she is often confined to the house, and she feels very isolated:

> '…it really gets me down. When you've gone from being completely active to suddenly losing so much, it tends to make you feel like you're not whole… I'm sitting here on my own 90 per cent of the time – the only people I see are Bill and Alexandra…'

However, parents emphasise that the advantages of employment depend on the sort of work that is both available and possible, and the support that has been put in place. They also point out that there is more to life than paid employment. Susie observes:

> 'Yes, work can be incredibly therapeutic, but there need to be things in place to help people, and quality of life shouldn't just be about you've got a job so you're entitled to a quality of life, quality of life should be for everybody…'

Parents highlight the complexity of balancing work and being a parent. Ginny comments:

> 'Work is good for you, depending what the work is…but if you have a family you still have to attend to children's needs and recover energies at the end of the day…'

Rose agrees:

'Work is good, if it's a job you like doing and it's reasonably well paid and it's not too stressful and it's not taking its toll on your health…and you've got support for your children.'

Families feel that the Government and personal advisers need to bear family responsibilities in mind when encouraging disabled people to access employment. As Rose points out:

'The Government need to look at the whole thing, the circumstances of family life, illness, what the Government can provide, what caring support is available…'

Ill-considered references to people 'languishing on benefits'[14] and 'benefits dependency'[15] and a sometimes vitriolic press campaign, have had an impact on parents' perceptions of the Government's welfare-to-work strategy. Families question whether the Government is motivated by a desire to improve the lives of disabled people or to save money. Amrit observes:

'All they're interested in is targets. They don't care about what sort of a dead-end job they put you into… You see these posters announcing 'We've got x amounts of people into employment' and you think 'Whoa', but how may of them left a job a day later?…They say 'We'll stay with you for two months', but what happens when you relapse?'

Employment services

Although families want more support to help them access employment, they are concerned that this is not always relevant or appropriate, and rarely leads to paid work. Disabled parents who are endlessly job searching become demoralised when they are repeatedly turned down for job interviews. Linda comments:

'When I think of the jobs I've written after and not had replies it's so disheartening…'

Some families are sceptical about new initiatives to help them access employment. Ginny reports:

'…various [private agencies funded by the DWP] have contacted me and said 'We're trying to get disabled people into employment and we can offer you rehabilitation and courses on computing'…I'm thinking 'What makes you the expert? I don't need a nurse, I need a job…' My own reaction to that is if you want me to work, offer me a job in your office doing this for other people who don't know how to find a job… If you don't have the skills to find a job, the chances are the jobs aren't there…'

Families welcome the support of their personal adviser. Bill observes that his personal adviser at Jobcentre Plus 'was a brilliant bloke, he was disabled himself…' However, they emphasise that personal advisers cannot force employers to give them a suitable job. Linda comments:

'My PA is very, very good and very helpful… She rings me up and tells me about what jobs there are, but [employers] don't want me because I don't have [the right qualifications].'

A number of parents with learning disabilities express frustration with the services provided by Jobcentre Plus. William comments '…they keep getting new people and there's no passing on of the information', Maria observes that people 'make assumptions' and Teresa reports that 'they have no respect, no respect. They don't listen to you, they say 'Oh she's got learning difficulties…''

Families feel frustrated that Jobcentre Plus sends them on endless courses, but does not find them jobs. Although Linda was very happy with a 'return-to-work' course she did at her local college that included computer skills, she became disheartened when it did not result in employment. 'It was a great course…if only you could get a job at the end…'

A number of parents with learning disabilities also question the relevance of the courses they are sent on. Teresa comments that when she was on jobseeker's allowance, she was told she had to go on a course. She asked if she could go on a catering course, but said that she did not mind what she did provided it was not computing. She was sent on a computing course.

Work and health

Official discussion has focused on the benefits that appropriate paid work – and an increase in income – may bring to disabled adults. However it is not this simple. Although most parents would like to work, they have concerns about the impact that balancing employment alongside their health and parental responsibilities could have on their health.

On the one hand, Susie acknowledges that being at home on her own would have been extremely difficult '...I most probably would have cracked up again because if you're on your own 24/7...' On the other hand, she reports that struggling to work full time for 20 years generated a number of breakdowns and hospital admissions. She feels that her mental health problems exacerbated difficulties working, and that working compounded her mental health problems:

> 'I was a person who would set these standards to show to yourself and everybody else that your illness doesn't dominate you and make you less of a worker...'

Susie's daughter, Anna, felt that access to a part-time, less stressful job would have mitigated the negative impact working had on her mother's health:

> 'I didn't want her at home all the time because I know she likes to be independent [but] if she got a job where the workload was less, then maybe she would be less stressed...'

Although part-time work is a welcome option, disabled parents emphasise that working fewer hours can still generate exhaustion and stress levels more usually associated with full-time employment. Louise comments:

> 'I really think we should be either paid the same amount to do fewer hours, or some adjustment, because it is exhausting... It's hard to get through your work day for many of us, let alone coming back and taking responsibility for the family.'

Although Amrit is keen to access paid employment, she is worried about the impact it might have on her mental health:

> 'At Jobcentre Plus they draw up this chart saying you'll be £120 a week better off – but is it likely to make me happier or is it likely to be a trigger [of mental health problems] for me – like becoming homeless was a trigger?... They seem to think if you're in a job you'll stay well. They say 'When you work you probably don't fall ill' – but I'm going to fall ill because it's biologi-

cal. I've been to college, I've still fallen ill. I've worked, I've still fallen ill –
getting £3,000 saved in my bank account isn't going to help when I fall ill.'

Louise highlights the difficulties of retaining employment when she developed a secondary impairment eight months ago, even though she worked for a large government agency. Although she was keen to retain her skilled and demanding professional job, she found handling new – and often faulty – special equipment extremely stressful:

> 'I struggled with so many new things – voice activated software, a headset for the phone…and then it didn't work, and I had to have a PA [personal assistant] as well as a driver, and I was dealing with an awful lot of pain, and I just couldn't cope with all of it any more.'

Barriers to employment

Stigma and discrimination

Although families welcome any support that will enable them to make a choice about employment, in the light of the discrimination disabled people experience on a daily basis, the parents interviewed thought it was unfair and unjust to pressurise them to access work. Until stigma and discrimination are eliminated within society as a whole, our interviewees do not hold out much hope of employers' attitudes changing.

Rose observes:

> 'There's legislation came out where you have to have access for disabled people, but you go up to the bank and I can't get in…it's got no ramp… [and at the supermarket] you have to fight for shopping trolleys…half an hour later we were still waiting for a porter to take it to the car…'

Lack of understanding about mental illness is viewed as a major problem. Susie comments:

> '[My employers] never really understood my illness…when I've gone back each time after a bleak time of illness I thought that I needed more support then than at any time, and they didn't understand quite how to do that… It was like 'Susie's back and away we go'. I think what I would have liked is

for somebody, my manager, to say 'Look, you've been really poorly, can you tell me something about how you feel, about what your illness is, and would you tell me something about what we could do to help you, would you like to pace your work differently or try and do something different, do you need things that are not going to be so stressful for you?' But it wasn't like that... so I would overcompensate then by pushing myself to hitting a top standard of achievement all the time – but that's a manic thing – that goes with the territory...'

Anna has strong – and informed – views about the lack of understanding displayed by her mother's employers:

'My mum's employers didn't support her or anything. Unless you walk in the shoes of the person, or walk in the shoes of somebody who is close to the person, you never really understand. I think the only thing you can do is make employers more aware of the fact that people with mental illness need support, but at the same time they shouldn't just view people with mental illness as people who aren't capable. I think my mum's very capable when she's well, but she doesn't need to get to the point where she's unwell...'

Given the general lack of awareness of mental health issues displayed by Anna's teachers and the often prejudiced approach adopted by her friends, she does not think that discrimination is likely to be eliminated in the near future:

'I've never once heard anything about mental illness be mentioned at school ever. It's just not talked about...'

Parents with learning disabilities experience high levels of discrimination and report that they are routinely overlooked when it comes to interviews for suitable jobs – 'they always give it to the next person.' On the few occasions they do get work, families report that they are sent to the lowest paid jobs, which are often not in their own areas.

Teresa reports that her daughter, who has Asperger's Syndrome, has also encountered problems accessing employment, although she has a degree, is proficient with computers and has attended endless interviews. When she lowered her sights and applied for a job shelf-filling at a local shop she was turned down on the grounds that they were 'cutting back on staff'. Parents comment that when it comes to giving them a job 'most places are cutting back.'

Louise feels that her (public sector) employer could have done much more to help her keep her job:

> 'The workload remained the same…they should have made more effort to re-deploy me…'

She reports that her over-worked colleagues displayed an understandable, but shocking, lack of awareness of her problems:

> 'I felt my colleague at the office couldn't understand…and these are highly educated people who are aware of these issues, they work with disabled people and older people… If only I could do it from home or work three days a week…'

Linda discusses the frustration of continuously applying for jobs and getting turned down or being left in limbo on 'reserve lists'. She reports:

> 'They have a national scheme to employ disabled people, but it doesn't seem to work… I had an interview with the tax office…they sent me to occupational health to see what I would be needing, but I'm still on the reserve list…'

Disabled parents – at least 50 per cent of whom are women – may not be able to undertake the sort of physically demanding part-time work that is available to non-disabled women. This renders it even more difficult to access jobs. Ginny, a disabled parent who runs a service user group, points out:

> 'Young mums could work at Tesco filling shelves, but this is not a suitable job for many disabled people. There needs to be differentiation…'

Linda comments:

> 'If I could, I would have gone into a factory or got a job waitressing, but I couldn't do it physically…'

Even when disabled people do get as far as an interview, they report that they are at a disadvantage if they have been out of employment for many years. When Linda was interviewed for a job with the tax office she observes:

'It was particularly stressful and hard...and some of the things they asked me – examples of problem solving... Not being in a workplace for a long time I had to think of other examples...'

Public attitudes can limit the sort of work a disabled adult can undertake. Amrit has self-harmed since she was a teenager. She comments:

'I've done work here and there, but it's difficult...for example, people freak out with my arms because I have horrendous scars – so Top Shop aren't going to say 'Come and work for us'... I try looking at it from their perspective – I say 'I'm well most of the time' [but] they're thinking, 'You're going to need that time off.' I could work for the first few weeks of a bad episode, or the last few weeks, but I need three, four or five weeks off during the really bad phases...'

Families report that support that has been put in place by the Government to help disabled people access employment can feel stigmatising. Amrit comments:

'Jobcentres have mental health advisers or lone parent advisers, or disability advisers – you have to choose which one you are... There's MENCAP saying 'Labels are for tins not for people' and there you have jobcentres saying 'mental health adviser', and you're standing in front of this sign, in front of other people...'

Skills, qualifications and training

As discussed in Chapter 1, disabled people are often likely to work well below their level of skills because they may face discrimination irrespective of their level of educational achievement. Such discrimination may occur because of the inflexibility of most employment structures and working environments, and because people may be unable to cope with the stress levels and long-hour culture often associated with professional employment opportunities. Louise comments:

'I'm desperate to get back to work, I know I have so much to offer. I have very specific and unusual skills and experience and I can't use them...the more professional you've been the harder it is – my skills are very particular [and] I couldn't work five days...'

Although she is willing to take on work at a lower level than she is used to, Louise is beginning to lose heart:

> 'The longer it goes on my confidence is sapping so fast. I know the rate of change, a new initiative, a document to absorb – and I feel I'm already out of date…'

Research also indicates that people who are disabled, and people who live in poverty, are less likely to get the qualifications they need to access well-remunerated employment.[16] The Government recognises that low skills and qualifications pose a barrier to employment, and has set up a number of training courses for disabled people. However, as discussed above, parents are not convinced that they will help. In a world in which qualifications are ever more important, disabled people may feel discriminated against because of interrupted schooling or difficulties gaining academic qualifications. Linda, who is 44, is frustrated by employers' obsession with qualifications: 'I've got the experience, but all they want is qualifications…'

Mental health problems during childhood and adolescence often disrupt studying and training. Susie reports:

> 'I had always been erratic at school, being a manic depressive you're like that, but it's hard to say whether it was an illness or that's the way it was. I never thought I had real problems until I was about 15, 16… I just thought it was my age, until it started going on and on… I did quite badly in my GCSEs…'

Combining training and parental responsibilities is difficult. Sally comments:

> '…doing a full-time degree and having a little boy was too much. I was living on campus. It was just too much to try and be a student and be a mum at the same time… I found myself turning into a monster. You either do one thing really well or you do two things badly…'

Amrit did not complete her academic training because of her mental health problems. She comments:

> 'My dream job is teaching, if I get my degree by the time I'm 30…but I don't know whether I'll be able to… As long as I remain well – but if they can't control my illness with medication I don't think I'll be able to do it.'

Some parents fear that they will be pushed into inappropriate jobs, irrespective of their skills or qualifications. Bill, who worked as a kitchen porter after being made redundant is hoping to retrain when his health improves:

> 'I've been used to doing engineering work – I'm not cut out to be a kitchen porter…'

Liz comments:

> 'I was always hoping to go back to work. As soon as the children were old enough to go to school, I went into the caring professions. I wanted to be an RGN [nurse]. I went on a day release course, and wanted to go on and train on a full-time basis…but I got my diagnosis that January…'

Constant rejections by prospective employers are demoralising and demeaning. Linda comments:

> 'I've been looking for work for ages, for over a year. It doesn't sound that long, but it seems like ages… It's demoralising. You get to the point you don't want to bother, you get doors shut in your face all the time. I'm an intelligent person, I've got a lot to offer. I wish they would look beyond the need for qualifications…'

Administrative barriers

Benefit and support services

The erratic and complex nature of the benefit system continues to pose major barriers to employment, as Rose points out:

> 'It takes a long time to get benefits put into place, and get to know what you're entitled to…say for example, it takes six to eight weeks to get benefits like income support and housing benefit… It was absolutely appalling when John came off work [to care for Steven]…it makes you think twice, it makes everybody think twice… When Steven went back into hospital I said to John 'Thank God you didn't go back to work because we would have had to been in the same situation again'

For parents with learning disabilities, the complexity of the benefits system undermines their confidence about applying for short-term jobs. Although a nine-month job that was suitable for someone with learning difficulties had come up the previous year, members of the group were worried about accessing benefits when the job came to an end: 'It's too much stress.' 'It makes you think.' 'At least benefits is safe money'.

Sick or disabled parents, who have had to fight for support at home, question whether appropriate support will be provided in the work-place. Rose comments:

> 'It's hard enough getting care in the home, how are they going to get care in the workplace?... If it's anything like my son trying to get statemented...'

The Access to Work scheme is designed to help employers with some of the costs of adapting workplaces to meet the needs of disabled workers. Although this scheme is clearly crucial, families report ongoing problems with its implementation. However, Louise reports that there is no financial support for pain or when people have to cut down from full-time to part-time work because of an impairment or disability. Her attempts to find a new job have been rendered difficult by cut-backs in the organisation that usually provides her with transport and which is funded by Access to Work. Although she is keen to attend an interview for a job, even though it is below her skill level, she does not know if she will be able to get there:

> 'The taxi fare is £100... If Access to Work don't provide it, the likelihood of local authority picking up the tab is inconceivable... I've had a bad time with Access to Work throughout – endless endless fights... I call it 'Access to Stress, or Access to Nothing'... Either they have it and fund it properly or they stop pretending...'

Disabled parents emphasise that their ability to work is directly linked with the provision of appropriate childcare – and not just during the day. Ginny comments:

> 'If you are disabled and you have a family, you still have to attend to the children's needs and recover your energies, and you're likely to be knackered at the end of the day...'

Employment and family life

Balancing employment alongside caring for children is difficult for all parents, but it is more demanding for sick or disabled parents. Although many disabled parents would welcome the opportunity to undertake some form of paid employment, it is problematic balancing employment alongside their caring responsibilities and health conditions. They fear that the additional stress could damage their health, undermine their ability to parent their children and put a strain on relationships.

A number of the parents interviewed are lone parents. They worry about their ability to care for their child and work. Amrit, who joined an employment agency which helps disabled people to access employment, explains:

> 'My criteria was so tight... I said I need a job within school hours... I'll be using public transport – I can't drive... I need to drop my daughter off at school and then get to wherever the job is. I'm not going to be there until 9.30 and I have to pick her up at 3.30 and I ask 'What about holidays and half-terms?' They say 'Have you got friends? Is there nobody to else to look after her for you?' But I'm a 'single being' – I don't have any family support, I'm completely on my own... My daughter goes to an inner-city school. I'm not happy about leaving her there for after-school clubs until 6.30 in the evening. Maybe if I lived in a nice area...'

Disabled lone parents who do work report that it impacts on their ability to parent. Susie says:

> 'I was always exhausted. I hadn't got the energy to work and be a parent, it was either/or, and I just thought I'm working. I'm making money. I'm paying my way – I thought one day Anna would be back with me...the guilt goes on for years and years and years, it's almost as destructive as having a mental illness... Home life impacts on your work and work impacts on your home life, it's a whole life...but there's no quality of life, there's no enjoying yourself...very, very stressful... Upon reflection, I think it would have been better to say 'Look, I've been really ill, I've had a breakdown, Anna is a priority...'

Lack of support with additional caring responsibilities also has an impact on the employment opportunities for non-disabled partners. Lily's husband, John, had to give up his job when their son Steven got leukaemia and was admitted to hospital. Rose, a wheelchair user, is unable to care for Steven when he is in hospital because of problems with access. She also has to care for her three older children. She comments:

> 'My husband is not disabled. He's able bodied and he's been employed since he was 16. However, he had to take time off to care for Steven, and he couldn't go back to work with Steven going to hospital every week... John's boss said you can come back to work, but they weren't happy for him to take time off to take Steven to hospital, me to hospital... Fair enough, let him go into work, but they have to provide me with carers and somebody to take Steven to hospital...'

Disabled parents who are primary carers (often, although not always, mothers) consider that they are at a greater disadvantage. Ginny observes:

> 'If a disabled person did not actually have to do practical childcare in the family they would have a higher chance of being able to promote their abilities. For example, I can write a letter, I can type, if I didn't have to also pace myself so that I could look after the children when they come back from school and do all the other things, I could go to work and write letters somewhere else... if I could depend on somebody to look after the children in the evening I would be able to do that job.'

The impact of employment on children

The Government emphasises that paid employment is in the best interest of children because it reduces levels of poverty. However, although many of the parents to whom we spoke would like to have the option of working, and would welcome additional income, they are worried that accessing paid employment might increase stress levels for both them and their children. Ginny does not think children's lives will be improved 'by forcing people into work' if the conditions of paid employment are not sufficiently flexible to enable parents with limited energy and other physical/mental constraints to balance work alongside their parental responsibilities.

Anna is delighted that her mother has given up full-time employment and that she can now live with her:

> 'I don't think that my mum should have gone on working as long as she did. I think that as soon as she felt that things were too much, she should have given up her job because although it would have meant that I wouldn't have got so

much because she would have had less money, I would have rather have seen her happy than see her so down…the stress and strain showed…'

The cost of employment

Disabled people incur additional costs that are directly related to impairment – for example, for extra heating, laundry and clothing, or special equipment. Furthermore, disabled people have to pay for personal support, goods and services, and help with tasks that non-disabled people can do for themselves.[17] Disabled parents emphasise that going to work generates additional disability-related costs for them as individuals, as well as for employers, and fear that a combination of being in low-paid work, working shorter hours and incurring additional costs might leave them worse off in work.

Anecdotal evidence indicates that moving into employment sometimes triggers a reassessment of disability living allowance (DLA), which is designed to help with the extra costs of disability. However, disabled parents point out that their care and mobility needs may actually go up when they move into paid employment. Ginny observes:

> 'You need the DLA mobility component to get you to work – without DLA or its equivalent I wouldn't have got into work in the first place…'

Low-paid work may leave disabled parents worse off because they have less time and energy to manage on an inadequate budget. Ginny comments:

> 'Disabled parents who are not in work can save money by having time, but you can't save money if you're at work on a low salary – particularly if you're disabled. Your choice of shop is restricted by how far you can go and your energy capacity. You may have to go to a closer shop that's more expensive if you're at work. Do you have to pay for somebody else to do something if you haven't got the energy to do it? Disabled people don't have the capacity to recover energy quickly… This is why there are so many disabled people out of work – the costs of it simply cannot be sustained with the salary that people are earning…'

There are other costs involved. As Sally comments:

> '...if you're sacrificing time spent with your very young child you need some compensations – but they're not necessarily better off... Because the work isn't skilled work, you're not gaining anything but money, but if it's not more money...'

The situation does not necessarily get better when children grow older. Although Ginny's daughter is at university and her younger son will be going to university next year, there are still problems with working:

> 'I have been offered a part-time job, but the additional income will be negligible when additional tax payments, loss of SDA [severe disablement allowance], and the increased loss of grant and tuition fee remissions are taken into account. I would have to take a full-time, well-paid job to make a positive impact on our finances, and I just don't have the stamina to cope with that type of load. I'd be off sick within a fortnight with exhaustion... There comes a point at which pacing oneself becomes more important than money, because it keeps people from complete collapse and out of hospital.'

Louise comments:

> 'The costs go up if you're disabled, but they're higher if you're working. You either need additional income or additional help... If you're so tired at the end of the day you're going to rely more and more on electricity and machines [such as dishwashers, washing machines, micro-waves etc]...'

Parents point out that the stress of working can generate extra costs to medical services. Anna comments:

> '...if [my mum] hadn't had so much pressure she wouldn't have been as ill as she was... The times she went into hospital were the times the work stress was the worst, so if she hadn't had so much work stress I don't think she would have had so many times when she had to go into hospital.'

Rose emphasises that disabled people are often carers and that if they move into employment, 'it's going to cost the Government more because they're going to have to care for the [disabled children or disabled adults] they look after...'

Caring responsibilities

Disabled parents sometimes have additional caring responsibilities over and above being a parent. Although statistics are thin on the ground (in *Improving the Life Chances of Disabled People* the Government reports that 'Some families will include disabled parents and disabled children although there is little specific data on this group')[18] a number of disabled parents report that they care for both sick or disabled adults and/or sick or disabled children, and that this impacts on their ability to undertake employment.

Rose, whose youngest child Steven has leukaemia, comments:

> 'If I got a job, well and good, but I cannot work because I have no support from the Government to provide care for my child because he doesn't fit in to any category... If we are to go out to work – they will have to pay some-body to come and look after my child...'

Susie, a lone parent, helped care for her terminally ill mother for some years. After her mother died, her father became ill and she had to care for him, but she reports that her caring responsibilities were never taken into consideration:

> 'If I was in crisis and needed to see the psychiatrist and get my pills, but nobody ever said 'Do you need support as a family, do you need somebody to help you do some of the caring, we know you're working?'...nobody ever asked that obvious question.'

Benefits

Given high levels of poverty among disabled people and the difficulties accessing paid employment, it is imperative that the benefit system is adequate. However, although the Government argues that it is committed to providing financial support for people who cannot work, the families we spoke to highlight a number of problems with the social security system.

Adequacy

The Government argues that incapacity benefit (IB) is just one part of a package of financial support for disabled people. This also includes DLA, which is intended to cover additional disability-related costs and can trigger disability premiums within income support and tax credits. Disability and carer organisations have long argued that extra-cost disability benefits do not cover the additional financial needs of disabled people and their carers. Furthermore, DLA does not take the additional costs of being disabled and being a parent into consideration – for example, the need for additional cleaning, transport, convenience foods and social excursions.[19]

Information

Accessing DLA is extremely difficult and take-up of DLA is low.[20] Families find it difficult accessing information about benefits. Rose observes:

> 'If you go the benefit office and say 'I'm disabled', they're not going to tell you basically what you're entitled to because half of them don't know...'

Susie comments:

> 'I didn't know how I would be if I gave up work. You don't know financially what the situation is. Nobody said to me 'You know, if you want to actually focus on being a parent there are things that can help you. There are benefits that enable you to have your child with you...'

Low take-up of disability benefits is viewed as an important issue. Linda observes:

> 'There's so much money that isn't being claimed – what are they doing to make sure that people are getting it? When you think of all the information about the pension credit, on the telly and in the papers, they don't do that for DLA...'

Incapacity benefit

Although the Government is concerned about the costs of IB, recipients report that moving from employment onto IB (which in April 2006 ranged from £59.20 to £78.50) results in a traumatic drop in income. Bill explains:

> 'We were on a very good wage before, and you tend to set your stall out to that level – but then you lose your house and you lose everything…'

Susie reports that moving out of work and onto IB was financially very difficult:

> 'I was on £20,000 a year and then I was on £3,500 a year… And every year you get a little bit more benefit money, but everything else goes up much more extremely – bills go up, everything goes up, so the benefit you get doesn't cover everything that's gone up, so you're a little bit worse off every year.'

Living on benefits is a constant struggle. Rose comments bitterly:

> '[The public] feel that these people who've been claiming benefits for a long time are getting a lot of money, but you don't get anything… We don't like to sponge off the Government. We feel guilty, but we haven't got a choice…'

Administration

Applying for benefits is stressful, difficult and often demeaning. A complex and impenetrable system means that families often do not get their full benefit entitlement.

Bill reports that it was not just losing his job and a good income that was a source of stress – applying for IB was a nightmare:

> 'There was one medical on top of another, they couldn't decide…the doctors were doubting my word from the word go…they make out you're always pulling the wool over their eyes…they're trying to trip you up all the time… Medical assessments are not very sensitive at all… You walk in there and you're made out to be a criminal and a fraud straight away…you shouldn't be treated like that…'

Families worry constantly that their benefits will be reduced or taken away. Rose asks:

> 'What do we do if this money stops? Will I say to my son who is dying, 'Sorry we can't come any more, they've stopped the money'?... You know, they can fine you or whatever, but who fines the Government?'

Gill, who facilitates a disabled parent group, explains that although the group was set up to provide support for people as parents, an enormous amount of time is spent discussing problems and issues around benefits. Parents in the group described the amount of time they spend trying to sort out their benefit claims, access emergency funds when their benefits do not come through, and discussing their needs with a huge array of officials who do not always display much understanding or sensitivity about learning disabilities: 'They were so nasty to us, I came out crying. They make you feel this small.' Families report that it is a full-time job to keep on top of things: 'It's a constant battle – especially when you don't understand the forms.' Two families in the group report that their benefits were stopped 'just before Christmas'. 'We had no food for the children – we had soup on Christmas day'. 'I had to get some emergency support. I applied for £50 – they gave me £25.'

Denise, who has learning disabilities, reported on the stress involved when her severely disabled son lost his DLA:

> 'They said he wasn't disabled – they took it away – we went weeks without benefits.'

The family was also thrown into crisis when her husband lost his IB just before Christmas in 2004. They were sent the wrong form to fill in (a first-time application form rather than a renewal). When they got the right form back they had five days to fill it in. Although they returned the form by special delivery – and checked it had arrived safely – the office claimed it had not arrived. When Denise's mother (who is a volunteer benefit adviser) contacted the IB office, she was told that all the files had been lost. Although the IB was reinstated at appeal in September 2005, it has yet to be paid.

Stigma

Although the incidence of disability benefit fraud is very low, families feel themselves to be under permanent scrutiny, not just from benefit officials and medical practitioners, but also from members of the public.

Liz and Bill feel anxious about people knowing that they are reliant on benefits. Liz comments:

> 'There are supposed to be a lot of concessions for people with low incomes and disabilities – but it's only £1 or 50p or less…and then you've got the embarrassment of providing the proof – you're in a queue with people looking over your shoulders… You feel put down all the time because you don't work – people look down on you, people call you low life…'

Liz and Bill's neighbour has recently reported them to the DWP for benefit fraud. Although a social security inspector has confirmed that they are entitled to their disability benefits, and advised them to take legal advice, they live in constant fear that they will lose their benefits.

Rose comments:

> 'We don't tell people we're on income support, we pretend we're in work. We don't want to be judged… People seem to think if you're on income support you're a scrounger and you don't want to work. People don't know the whole situation, but why should we have to explain?…'

Disabled people who receive benefits often feel that if they undertake any activity – even if it is good for their health – they will lose their entitlement. As Liz comments:

> 'The stupid thing is you've only got to do something on a regular basis, they think you're doing something you shouldn't be doing…'

Rose enjoys horse riding, but doing so has generated a certain amount of criticism:

> 'I've ridden in the past, it makes a huge difference, but lots of people say 'If you ride a horse why do you need so much help?'…but it improves me in quite a few ways… It's nice to know that I can still do things…'

Impact on children

Living on an inadequate income has an impact on children. Susie, who has given up work so she can spend more time with her daughter explains:

> 'You do adjust because you get used to going without, but I do get upset if I can't get something for Anna, that she should not ever suffer because I'm mentally ill and had to give up my job. It's not her fault, and she shouldn't be having a second-class life… Sometimes there have been trips at school where she would quite like to go, and I have to say 'Well, that's quite a lot of money and we would have to go into major debt', and Anna says 'Well, it's not that important' – but if we could have afforded it she would have wanted to go.'

Gill explains that the parents with learning disabilities who attend the group are very resourceful: 'They start buying Christmas presents in October…' However, parents in the group report that it is a struggle surviving on benefits. They worry about their children. 'They don't have things other children have'. 'The kids can't have shoes.' 'They just get bits and pieces – we never buy them new clothes, people give us clothes – the children don't like it though…' Maria comments:

> 'Our son wants to go to France [with the school] but it's going to cost £154 – I had to say no.'

Susie would not be able to cope without the financial support of her family. However, a number of families are not in touch with their extended families and have to cope on their own. Amrit comments:

> '…there is no family infrastructure or support – I really am a single person…'

Moving onto benefits is often associated with severe housing problems. Liz and Bill struggled to buy their council home in order to attain some level of long-term financial security, but when Bill moved onto IB they could not keep up with the mortgage payments and they lost their house:

> 'We had to give up the house, we were threatened with B&B… Alexandra was a year old, Judith was 10…'

Services

The provision of appropriate support services is crucial to enable families to cope and stay together. However, families report that lack of coherent and sensitive supportive services, and the tendency to treat individual members of the family differently depending on whether they are a child, an adult or a carer, undermine the efficacy of statutory services, and compound the day-to-day stress involved in coping with a disability or health problem and in being a parent. Poor service provision increases costs and continues to have a negative impact upon disabled people's lives. Susie comments bitterly:

> 'The services don't fit people's lives, they don't even acknowledge that people have lives…'

Amrit reports:

> 'You're either too old, too young… There are too many things working against you…'

Although a number of documents and policy initiatives emanating from various government departments emphasise the importance of assessing disabled adults' parenting responsibilities,[21] families report that these are usually ignored. Amrit comments:

> 'The professionals around us don't see me as a mother… They see me as a 23-year-old Asian adult with mental health problems…they don't see the impact it has on my daughter.'

Susie reports:

> 'The hospital took quite good care of me…but I never sat down with the psychiatrists or the nurses. They never said 'What do you need to help you…to get more support in looking after your daughter so you could be with your daughter more… Unless I spoke about Anna she wasn't spoken about…'

Additional caring responsibilities, for parents as well as children, are sometimes overlooked. Susie reports:

'I was having to fight for my own rights and my father's rights…'

Although health practitioners are at the heart of the revised assessment process, families question whether they are the best people to assess their capability to work. Susie comments:

'The Government say 'Right, you go and see your GP – it's about time you go back to work, it's really good for you', but they can't help you into the right environment to get the support you need…'

The Green Paper relies heavily on decision makers to stream disabled people on the basis of evidence from a variety of medical practitioners. But disabled parents report that medical practitioners do not always agree:

'Now the Government are saying 'We've got to assess you to see if you can go out to work.' But how much does a person have to be pulled, and prodded and poked and questioned?… How can they separate people out?… I was under a GP, then you're under a neurologist, a cardiologist, you can add in a couple more [Ear Nose and Throat] people…and they're all telling you different things…'

Impact on children

A number of parents express concern that lack of support for their own needs results in them making additional demands on their children. Ginny reports:

'The main thrust of what disabled parents need is to support them as adults in their parenting role, rather than to label their children as 'in need', which requires ongoing supervision and assessment of the parent's capacity to parent their children – which is often no more appropriate than for parents who are not disabled…'

Rose reports that her older children have had to help care for her because her husband spends a lot of overnight stays in hospital with Steven. She observes:

'They never have a childhood – always caring for somebody… They have to grow up very, very quickly…they're doing jobs they shouldn't be doing. I find it quite abusive putting these kids through it because the Government won't provide care...'

Louise reports that:

'...I lean heavily on the rest of my family in a way that has been stressful for them. The girls – it's hard for me to decide what is reasonable for them – they have to help with cooking, but they have a lot of homework...'

Lack of support for their own care needs means that children sometimes miss out on everyday experiences. Liz comments:

'It's difficult to have Alexandra's friends over from school. If she has friends over they want to do things...'

A message to the Government

The families who participated in this small study provide some important messages for the Government. Although families believe that they have valuable skills and experiences, they highlight a number of concerns about the current system and the proposed changes and indicate which areas need much greater attention from policy makers.

Employment

Families recognise that paid employment can bring significant psychological and financial advantages – and many want to work. However, they do not feel that it is appropriate to bring more pressure to bear on disabled people to access work when they already want to do so. Linda comments:

'It's not the incentives. People like me are trying hard and not getting anywhere... I don't need to find work, but I do want to be useful... If I was working I'd probably be £20 a week better off – I'd lose some housing, but I would get a bit more money. I wouldn't mind about the £20 it's for me, I want to help, I want to contribute something...'

Disabled people should not be compelled to access paid employment – those who are willing and able to work should be provided with the support they need to do so. Those who cannot work should be provided with financial support that safeguards them and their children from poverty.

Barriers to employment

Families highlight a wide range of barriers to employment, including stigma and discrimination within society as a whole and among employers in particular, the inadequacies of the Access to Work system, difficulties gaining appropriate levels of qualifications and skills, and additional problems balancing employment with parental and caring responsibilities. Susie comments:

> 'We need to see employers who understand the variety of issues they may have to deal with. We need somebody to liaise with that person so if they're getting grotty they've got somebody to go and talk to…'

Government initiatives need to recognise that disabled parents face additional barriers to employment. More work should be done to reduce discrimination in the labour market, and parenting and caring responsibilities must be taken into consideration during the assessment process.

Low-paid work

Disabled parents – many of whom are lone parents – are concerned about the type of work available. They worry that they will be forced to participate in paid employment that may be part time, low paid, or stressful and unrewarding. A recent report issued by the Commission on Women and Work indicates that women, who are more likely to work part time in low paid employment because of 'taking time out of the labour market or reducing their working hours to care for children or other relatives',[22] continue to be disadvantaged in the workplace. They are significantly more disadvantaged if they are disabled. Families are concerned that accessing low-paid employment will not help their children. Ginny comments:

> '[The Government] could put somebody on an income bracket to let them get help to look after their children better than if they were simply on benefit…'

Increasing rates of employment among disabled parents will only help lift more children out of poverty if jobs are adequately paid and sustainable. Encouraging or compelling disabled parents to move into low-paid jobs will undermine official objectives on increasing employment and reducing child poverty.

Costs of employment

Although many disabled parents would like to be in paid employment, they emphasise that working is more costly for them – not just because they incur additional disability-related costs (such as travel and extra care needs), but in terms of family relationships and their own health. Disabled parents worry that balancing already complex lives alongside paid work may also have a negative impact on their ability to parent their children.

The additional costs of employment must be taken into con-sideration during the assessment process when deciding whether employment is appropriate or how it may be supported. If not, it is unlikely to be sustained.

Work-focused activities

Although families want more support to help them access employment, they are concerned that the advice and training given are not always rele-vant or appropriate, and rarely lead to paid employment. Although the support of their personal advisers is valued and welcome, families point out that they cannot oblige employers to give them a job. Disabled par-ents who are actively seeking employment report that courses run by Jobcentre Plus may not be relevant and do not always result in paid employment. Endlessly job searching without success is demoralising.

Parental responsibilities must be taken into consideration when drawing up action plans. Endless work-search activities may undermine disabled parents' ability to parent their children.

Benefit adequacy

Although families welcome the support that has been put in place to help disabled people – for example, disability premiums within income support and tax credits – they highlight a number of problems with the current benefit system, which have not been addressed by the proposed changes. These include poor information provision, low take-up of disability benefits, ineffective administration of the benefit and tax credit systems, and stigma. Families believe that more effort should go into ensuring that people get the benefits to which they are entitled. They question whether the proposals will improve the assessment process.

The Government needs to ensure that disabled people receive the disability benefits to which they are entitled, and that benefit levels safeguard parents and children from poverty.

Service provision

Families emphasise that fragmented services impose additional costs and undermine their ability to access paid employment. They point out that welfare reform programme and assessment procedures do not consider a disabled person's parenting responsibilities when assessing her/his ability to seek employment or deciding what additional care is needed at work and at home.

Disabled parents highlight the difficulties of balancing their health needs or disability alongside their parental responsibilities. Many disabled parents have additional caring responsibilities. Given the difficulties they have accessing help at home, they are sceptical about the chances of receiving the additional support they need to access paid employment.

Disabled parents do not just need support to help them access and retain employment, they need additional support for them and their children at home.

User involvement

Families highlight the importance of consulting disabled parents themselves when formulating policy. However, while *Fair Access to Care Services* stipulates that 'Councils should ensure that individuals are active partners in the assessment of their needs' and emphasises that 'Councils should recognise that individuals are the experts on their own situation and encourage a partnership approach to assessment', families are concerned that this approach is lacking in the Green Paper. Ginny comments:

> 'When they come to assessing people...they should also be looking at the sort of criteria in the *Fair Access to Care* document produced by the Department of Health[23] which requires that a disabled person should

be supported to undertake their social role – and that includes raising children…'

Families feel that they are the experts, and that they should be effectively and meaningfully consulted about policies that affect both them and their children.

Notes

1 Department for Work and Pensions, *A New Deal for Welfare: empowering people to work*, The Stationery Office, 2006

2 See H Stickland, Background paper for the HMT/DWP seminar 'Disabled Parents and Employment', 24 November 2003

3 HM Treasury, *Child Poverty Review*, The Stationery Office, 2004, published as part of the Spending Review 2004, reports that: 'There are around one million workless, disabled parents. A significant proportion say they would like to work.' (p22). The recently published *Improving the Life Chances of Disabled People* reports that: 'Among workless households with children the majority have at least one disabled parent…' It confirms that 'a quarter of children living in poverty have long-term sick or disabled parents.' (pp46 and 83)

4 HM Treasury, *Child Poverty Review*, The Stationery Office, 2004, p61

5 See note 4, p46

6 Department for Work and Pensions, *Households Below Average Income 1994/95-2004/05*, Corporate Document Services, 2006, Tables 4.4 and 4.7 show that before housing costs, of 2.4 million poor children, 26 per cent (around 624,000) were both income poor and recorded as living in a household with one or more disabled adult. The risk of income poverty for this group is 31 per cent (against an average risk for all children of 19 per cent).

7 See note 6, p22

8 T Burchardt, 'Barriers to Employment for Disabled Parents: the double whammy', paper delivered to HMT/DWP seminar 'Disabled Parents and Employment', 24 November 2003

9 J Casebourne and L Britton, *Lone Parents, Health and Work*, DWP Research Report 214, Department for Work and Pensions, 2004

10 See note 2

11 J Morris, *The Right Support: report on the task force on supporting disabled adults in their parenting role*, Joseph Rowntree Foundation, 2003

12 Department of Health, *Fair Access to Care Services: guidance on eligibility criteria for adult social care*, 2003

13 See note 4, p83

14 Used by Tony Blair in a speech in Hungary, 15 February 2004

15 A phrase which peppers the Green Paper, see note 1

16 See G Palmer, J Carr and P Kenway, *Monitoring Poverty and Social Exclusion*, Joseph Rowntree Foundation and New Policy Institute, 2005

17 See, for example, N Smith, S Middleton, K Ashton-Brooks, L Cox and B Dobson with L Reith, *Disabled People's Costs of Living: 'more than you would think?'*, The Policy Press for Joseph Rowntree Foundation, 2004

18 See Cabinet Office, Prime Minister's Strategy Unit, *Improving the Life Chances of Disabled People*, 2005 (a joint report with the Department for Work and Pensions, Department of Health, Department for Education and Skills and Office of the Deputy Prime Minister), p103, footnote 140 and note 12

19 See, for example, G Preston, *Family Values: disabled parents, extra costs and the benefit system*, Disability Alliance, 2004

20 Although there are no recent figures on take-up of DLA, estimated take-up of DLA care component is between 30 per cent and 50 per cent and take-up of DLA mobility component is estimated to be between 50 per cent and 70 per cent. See P Craig and M Greenslade, *First Findings from the Disability Follow-up to the Family Resources Survey*, Research Summary 5, HMSO, 1998

21 See note 18

22 Women and Work Commission, *Shaping a Fairer Future*, 2006 states that 'women are crowded into a narrow range of lower-paying occupations, mainly those available part time that do not make the best of their skills… Women returning to the labour market after time spent looking after children often find it difficult to find a job that matches their skills.' (p1)

23 See note 12

Five
Incapacity benefit and welfare reform
Gabrielle Preston

Introduction

This chapter considers the Government's proposals for the reform of inca-pacity benefits contained in the Green Paper, *A New Deal for Welfare: empowering people to work*. It is an edited, amended and updated ver-sion of the submission CPAG presented to the Work and Pensions Committee during its inquiry and written prior to the publication of the Green Paper in February 2006, and of CPAG's response to the Green Paper itself.[1] It summarises CPAG's views on welfare reform.

The reforms outlined in the Green Paper are designed to:

> ...break down the barriers that prevent many from fulfilling their potential, barriers that impede social mobility and, through worklessness and eco-nomic inactivity, consign people to poverty and disadvantage. (p2)

The Government hopes to reduce the number of people on incapacity benefits by one million by:

> ...increasing the number of people who remain in work when they fall sick or become disabled; increasing the number leaving benefits and finding employment; and better addressing the needs of all those who need extra help and support. (p24)

Central to the Green Paper is the desire:

> ...to reduce the number of people moving onto the new benefit, increase the number leaving benefit quickly, and better address the needs of those on the benefit, including additional payments to the most seriously disabled people. (p29)

The Green Paper: a summary of proposals

- Incapacity benefit (IB) and the disability premium within income support will be replaced with a new employment and support allowance (ESA) which 'focuses on how we can help people into work and does not automatically assume that because a person has a significant health condition or disability they are incapable of work…' (p41)
- People will need to satisfy a revised personal capability assessment before they become eligible for the employment or support component of the new allowance.
- Until a decision has been made about the severity of a person's disability and her/his ability to undertake work-related activities, s/he will be placed on a basic allowance, set at the jobseeker's allowance rate (£57.45 a week for most single adults in April 2006).
- A 12-week assessment process, including going through a revised personal capability assessment, will not focus on the 'nature of the specific illness or disability the individual has, but on the severity of the impact of that condition on the individual's ability to function.' (p39)
- People who are designated as able to undertake work-focused activities will be placed on the employment component of ESA. These claimants will be able to increase the basic allowance by attending work-focused interviews and 'taking steps to get them back in the market.'
- 'For people with the most severe functional limitations, it would be unreasonable to expect that they engage in work-related activity' (p39) and they will be placed on the support component of ESA. They will not be expected to engage in work-focused activities or to seek employment, although they may choose to do so. However, they will have to attend the initial compulsory work-focused interview eight weeks after claiming (as they do now in the Pathways to Work pilot). The new benefit will provide a higher level of financial support than is currently available via IB.
- Claimants will, as now, have a right of appeal at appropriate points in the decision making process. (p44)

The Government proposes to implement 'reform of the gateway, improvements to workplace health, increased support for claimants and removal of the perverse incentives in the system' and argues that this should 'significantly reduce the number claiming incapacity benefits.'[2]

This chapter asks whether these proposals are likely to improve the life chances and economic wellbeing of disabled people and considers whether they will improve or have a negative impact on outcomes for children. It asks whether work is an effective route out of poverty for everyone. Drawing on the experience of CPAG's welfare rights work, it considers whether the proposed changes will improve the administration and adequacy of the benefit system, or whether increased complexity will impose an untenable burden on an already unwieldy and often unjust system. It raises concerns about imposing increased conditionality and benefit sanctions on groups of people who are already vulnerable to poverty, and questions whether welfare reform is possible without addressing benefit adequacy.

This chapter views the Government's welfare reform proposals from a child poverty perspective. It considers whether the different sections in the Green Paper complement or impede each other, and whether they are informed by or undermine other policy initiatives instigated by the Government. It asks whether the Green Paper reflects and reinforces the recommendations and policy initiatives outlined in *Every Child Matters*,[3] the *Child Poverty Review*[4] and *Improving the Life Chances of Disabled People*.[5] It assesses whether it gives due weight to parenting responsibilities, family needs and income adequacy and whether it reflects a holistic, 'joined-up' approach to welfare reform. It also asks whether the proposals provide a coherent package of reform for families and children, or whether welfare reform will prove to be a costly and ineffective diversion.

The first part of this chapter sets out the contextual framework for the reform, and assesses its possible impact on disabled parents and their children. The second part considers the proposals outlined in the Green Paper. It also examines welfare delivery and benefit simplification, and assesses how these interact with the proposals on helping sick and disabled people. The chapter concludes with a number of recommendations.

Disability and employment

Disabled people are significantly more likely to live in poverty than non-disabled people because they are less likely to be in paid employment, are more likely to be in part-time or low-paid employment, are more likely to be reliant on benefits, and incur additional disability-related costs. People who are poor are also more likely to become sick or disabled. For example, the risk of developing a mental illness is around 25 per cent in the poorest fifth of the population – twice the rate for people on average incomes.[6] High levels of poverty are caused and exacerbated by inadequate or unreliable financial support, discrimination and fragmented service provision.

A number of factors are closely linked with disability:

- **Low income**. Although the Government accepts that disability is a cause of poverty, much less is made of the fact that living on a low income increases the risk of disability – although this is startlingly borne out by extensive research on health inequalities.[7]
- **Worklessness**. Of those children living in poverty who live in a workless household, just over half have at least one disabled parent. Of all workless couple households with children, two-thirds have at least one disabled parent.[8]
- **Poor working conditions**. An increase in conditions such as stress, depression and anxiety[9] suggests a link between being in low-paid, low-status occupations and the onset of sickness or disability.
- **Social and educational disadvantage**. The Prime Minister's Strategy Unit reports that:

  Low incomes, non-employment, and low education all independently increase the probability of someone becoming disabled. Many of these risk factors are amenable to policy intervention. Often the onset of ill-health or disability deepens pre-existing disadvantage.[10]

- **Educational disadvantage**. A recent report reveals that having no educational qualifications raises the odds of the onset of disability by over 55 per cent, which then greatly increases the risk of being out of work or in low-paid employment.[11]

The Green Paper recognises the barriers to employment faced by disabled people, accepts that they need additional support to access jobs and acknowledges the importance of providing more adequate financial support to those disabled adults who are unable to work. All these elements are crucial if child poverty is to be halved by 2010 and eradicated by 2020.

However, as discussed in Chapter 1, the recently published *Monitoring Poverty and Social Exclusion*[12] provides a depressing picture of the disadvantages disabled people face in the labour market in the UK and demonstrates the challenge faced by policy makers. Compared to non-disabled adults, disabled adults are more likely to be income poor, with the risk having risen over recent years. At any given level of qualification, disabled adults are likely to 'lack but want work'; nearly half of all disabled people of working age are economically inactive compared with only 15 per cent of their non-disabled counterparts.[13] Three-quarters of all working-age people who receive one of the key out-of-work benefits for two years or more are sick or disabled. Of those sick or disabled people in this position, one-third are aged 55 to retirement, one-third aged 45 to 54, and one-third are aged under 45.[14] *Monitoring Poverty and Social Exclusion* concludes that the fact that:

> At every level of qualifications, disabled people are both more likely to be low paid and more likely to be wanting but lacking work shows that the problem cannot lie solely with disabled people themselves...[this situation] can only arise if employers perceive disabled employees differently from non-disabled ones...this is evidence that the labour market effectively discriminates against disabled people.[15]

The TUC points out that 45 per cent of people who moved from incapacity benefit (IB) onto jobseeker's allowance (JSA) were still on benefit a year later (compared with only 28 per cent when non-disabled people were included). This highlights the very real difficulties disabled people still experience accessing employment and moving off benefit.[16]

Given these barriers to employment, work is too often an unreliable and unrealistic route out of poverty for many disabled people.

Disability and child poverty

Children with disabled parents

As discussed in Chapter 2, children with a disabled parent are disproportionately likely to be poor. The recently published *Households Below Average Income* (HBAI) statistics indicate that after housing costs have been accounted for, 24 per cent of the 3.4 million poor children in Great Britain (around 816,000) lived with one or more disabled adult in 2004/05. The risk of income poverty for this group was two in five (against an average risk for all children of 27 per cent). We also know the following:

- There are around 1.7 million disabled parents (some of whom live with other disabled parents), with around 2.2 million children in their care. Around 12 per cent of all parents are disabled, and 17 per cent of children have at least one disabled parent.[17] Disability and lone parenthood are also linked. One-quarter of lone parents have a long-standing illness or disability.[18]
- Nearly 840,000 – or 40 per cent (after housing costs) – of the 2.1 million children with disabled parents are living in poverty.[19]
- Like all disabled people, disabled parents face barriers to employment. While couples with children where neither is disabled have an employment rate of 97 per cent, this drops to 78 per cent when at least one of the couple is disabled. For non-disabled lone parents, the employment rate is almost 60 per cent, for disabled lone parents it is almost 40 per cent.[20]

Clearly meeting the needs of disabled parents is critical if the Government is to meet its targets to move one million people off incapacity benefits over the next 10 years, and to lift a further million children out of poverty by 2010. But is the Green Paper likely to draw disabled parents and their children out of poverty, or could increased conditionality and the threat of benefit sanctions have an adverse impact on the most vulnerable groups of parents, such as those with mental health problems, learning disabilities or fluctuating conditions?

Disability and lone parents

Children living in lone-parent households (many of which are also affected by disability and ill-health) also face a significant risk of living in poverty. Recent findings from the 2004 Families and Children Study reveal that lone parents, who account for around one-quarter of families with dependent children, are consistently worse off than couple families, and are twice as likely to describe their health as 'not good' compared with mothers in couple families.[21] One Parent Families reports that lone parents not only experience higher levels of poor health than other family types, but 26 per cent have a sick or disabled child.[22]

Lone parents are not only more susceptible to poverty and ill-health, but research indicates that the stress and strain of coping with disability without adequate support also takes its toll on relationships.[23] This needs to be recognised and addressed in the proposals on welfare reform.

Disabled children

Families with disabled children are disproportionately susceptible to poverty. Government statistics indicate that, in terms of income poverty, 30 per cent of children in households with a disabled child are living below 60 per cent of median income (after housing costs) compared with 27 per cent of households with no disabled children. This rises to 37 per cent if there is a disabled adult in the household.[24] However, as discussed in Chapter 3, statistics underestimate the incidence of poverty because they include disability benefits as income but take no account of additional costs and, therefore, overestimate the incomes of households affected by disability.

The need to care for a disabled child limits the hours a parent can work: only 3 per cent of mothers with disabled children are in full-time employment (compared with 22 per cent of mothers with non-disabled children) and only 13 per cent manage part-time work (compared with 39 per cent of mothers with non-disabled children).[25] Any reform of the welfare system must address the particular needs of families with disabled children.

The Green Paper reports that the new cross-government Office for Disability Issues will 'act as focal point within government and drive forward the implementation of the overall strategy' (p49) and cites *Improving the Life Chances of Disabled People* recommendations to 'improve support for families with young disabled children' and help 'a smooth transition into adulthood by, for example, removing 'cliff edges' in service provision' (p49). In the next section we assess whether the Green Paper accords with these aspirations.

The Green Paper: a response

The proposals outlined in the Green Paper on incapacity benefits are significant and complex. They have many ramifications at both a wider policy, and a detailed administrative, level. The implications of the changes for other entitlements are under-explored and CPAG will continue to raise questions on these: clarifying the relationship between the new employment and support allowance (ESA) with other benefits will be crucial as legislation is prepared.[26] This section focuses on the policy issues that emerge, outlines CPAG's views on what is being proposed and discusses some of the detailed proposals outlined in the Green Paper.

Employment

The benefits of work for individuals, and for the economy, are at the heart of the Green Paper, which argues that employment is 'good for individuals, good for families, good for communities and good for Britain.' (p21)

The labour market

The Government reports that there has been an overall fall of around one million in the number of jobless people on benefits, and that the biggest improvement has been 700,000 fewer people claiming unemployment benefit. Such figures are encouraging, but it is hard to know how the Government will move one million disabled people off incapacity benefits at a time when unemployment is starting to rise and, according to recent reports, is 'likely to hit one million by the summer after the latest sharp rise in joblessness took the total to its highest level in two and a half years'.[27]

Quality of jobs and in-work poverty

The Green Paper categorically states 'the problem is not a lack of jobs.' (p18) However, many disabled people disagree. The Pathways to Work pilots increased the number of disabled people leaving IB by 8 per cent.[28] However, there is little evidence about the kind of jobs people have accessed. The Government agrees that low quality jobs have an adverse impact on people's health. In 1999, the Health and Safety Executive estimated that work-related stress cost employers at least £353 million a year and cost society at least £3.7 billion.[29] The Department of Health reports that:

> A lack of job control, monotonous and repetitive work, and an imbalance between effort and reward are associated with a higher risk of coronary heart disease and other health problems...[30]

> Although work is generally good for people's health, poor health and safety management increases the risk of occupational disease and injury. 'Bad' jobs may make people ill.[31]

People need to be reassured that there are flexible and well-paid jobs available, and that they will be helped to build up their skills and progress at work. Furthermore, as shown in Chapter 4, some disabled parents report that balancing paid work alongside their health needs and family responsibilities may have a negative impact on their ability to parent.

In-work poverty is also an issue: 54 per cent of poor children live in a household with one or more parent in work.[32] We have particular concerns about disabled people, many of whom may have been seriously disadvantaged by the educational system and continue to be disadvantaged in the labour market, being 'encouraged' (or pushed) to participate in paid employment that may be part time, low paid, or stressful and unrewarding. This will not protect them from poverty and may damage their health or worsen their disability. We fear that this may be exactly the kind of employment that disabled people are likely to access if compelled to seek work. Encouraging people to access poorly paid employment may reduce the direct cost of IB to the Government in the short term, but it will not significantly increase the incomes of some of the UK's most disadvantaged groups and may generate increased costs in the long term both to individuals and to society because of worsening health. Poorly paid work is not a route out of poverty.

It is imperative that the Government monitors not only the number of disabled people moving into employment, but the sort of jobs different groups of disabled people access, and whether they are sustainable and can draw people out of poverty.

Barriers to employment

Employers

The Green Paper argues that 'the current system fails to engage with employers or to use them to channel more and better jobs towards disadvantaged people.' (p19) However, there is little evidence that employers are always prepared to give well-remunerated, rewarding jobs to sick and disabled people – particularly people with mental health problems or learning disabilities – and little indication that the Green Paper will improve this situation.

The fact that employers, who, like many other people in society, may feel unsure about working with disabled people and lack the confidence and knowledge to do so, continue to discriminate against them is borne out by the statistics reported in *Monitoring Poverty and Social Exclusion* (discussed above).

Employers must accept more responsibility for the low levels of employment among disabled people. There should be stronger requirements for them to make appropriate adjustments to assist disabled people to access work. It is unjust and inappropriate to expect disabled people to engage in endless work-focused activities if these are unlikely to lead to employment.

Mental health problems

The Government recognises that people with mental illness face significant barriers accessing paid employment. The Social Exclusion Unit report, *Mental Health and Social Exclusion*, acknowledges that 'adults with long-term mental health problems are one of the most excluded groups in society.'[33] According to the Unit, over 900,000 people claim sickness and disability benefits for mental health conditions. This group accounts for 40 per cent of all disabled people and is 'now larger than the total number of unemployed people claiming jobseeker's allowance in England.'[34] Despite the implementation of the Disability Discrimination Act, employers may find it difficult to employ someone with mental health problems, or to rehabilitate employees who experience the onset of problems. According to the Chartered Institute of Personnel and Development, one in five employers will not employ someone with mental health problems.[35]

Education and skills

The Green Paper recognises the need to 'improve the skills of individuals within these client groups to enable them to progress once they are in work' (p10) and accepts that 'the scale of the challenge is typically more concentrated in some of the poorest and most disadvantaged areas, and among people who often face other disadvantages such as low skills.' (p26) The Green Paper does not, however, discuss skills policy in any detail. Disabled people with low skills, who face multiple barriers to employment, will be expected to engage in work-focused activity. This needs to be more effectively linked with well-resourced skills initiatives that can assist people into sustained employment.

Although much is made in the Green Paper about increasing the expectations of disabled people, while the aspirations of disabled 16-year-olds are similar to those of their non-disabled counterparts, they are still disadvantaged in both the educational system and the labour market. By the time they are 18, 48 per cent of disabled young people will receive the equivalent of NVQ level 1 or below (equivalent of GCSE D-G or below). By the time they are 26, they are nearly four times as likely to be unemployed or involuntarily out of work than non-disabled people.[36] Improvements in education and training are an essential pre-requisite for improving employment levels among disabled people.

Childcare

The Government accepts that the provision of adequate, accessible and affordable childcare is fundamental to increasing the employment rate among lone parents. The ability of disabled people to engage in work-focused activities and to access employment is also directly linked with the availability of appropriate and accessible childcare (and transport). Although childcare is considered in the Green Paper in the section on lone parents, it has been largely ignored in the proposals for disabled people, highlighting one of its inconsistencies.

In the section on lone parents, the Green Paper reports that the Organisation for Economic Co-operation and Development believes that 'once employment and childcare support is available on a comprehensive basis, it would be reasonable to oblige sole parents on income support to make use of it'. (p57) However, despite improvements to childcare provision, it is not necessarily available, accessible, affordable or – in some cases – very good. Even if the Government doubled its current commitment of £6.5 billion (0.54 per cent of gross domestic product)[37] a year to finance childcare, it would still be half that spent by some other countries. *Opportunity for All* reports that 'Sweden and Finland invest heavily in childcare, spending 1.4 per cent and 0.9 of gross domestic product respectively.'[38]

There are other problems with childcare. Despite the increase to 80 per cent of covered costs in April 2006, the childcare element of working tax credit (WTC) has significant limitations. Take-up is low, the levels of support do not cover the often prohibitive costs, particularly in London and for disabled children, and the more disadvantaged families are least likely to access it.[39] The restrictive nature of current childcare support does not reflect family needs. Disabled parents may need access to child-care for some time before starting work, or to recoup the energy and con-fidence required to access employment. Continuity of childcare is in the best interest of children if employment breaks down, but the tax credit system does not support this.

Although government research indicates that children from disad-vantaged backgrounds derive most benefit from high quality childcare, CPAG is concerned that such children, who are more likely to be in work-less households and whose parents do not qualify for WTC, are likely to be excluded from provision. It is regrettable that the Green Paper does not address the childcare needs of disabled parents. We urge the Department for Work and Pensions (DWP), the Treasury and the Department for Education and Skills to ensure these agendas are joined up to support each other.

Parents should not be compelled to access employment if they have concerns about the quality and cost of the childcare available or if they need to spend time with their children. Such decisions should be respected, whether they are in or out of paid work.

Costs of employment

The Government recognises that employing disabled people may some-times generate additional costs for employers. The Access to Work scheme provides vital financial assistance for employers who need to make adjustments to the workplace. However, as discussed in Chapter 4, this is poorly publicised and not always efficiently administered.

Working generates extra costs for disabled people themselves. Although they rely on disability living allowance (DLA) to cover additional care and mobility costs (and the DWP has assured CPAG that 'there is no legal requirement for a DLA recipient to notify a return to or com-mencement of working'[40]), anecdotal evidence indicates that moving into employment sometimes triggers a reassessment of DLA which is often removed. This may leave people actually worse off if they access work. Substantial demands for repayments of 'overpaid' DLA following a re-assessment generate considerable emotional and financial stress.

We are concerned that some disabled people who are willing and able to work are unable to do so because the costs involved are untenable. The reassessment and/or removal of DLA when they access employment, and the recovery of alleged 'overpayments'

incurred in this way places disabled people under considerable stress and may render employment unfeasible.

Benefits

Adequacy

Much is made in the Green Paper about the role and the inadequacy of the benefits system. It reports that the 'welfare state has never been more important for economic success and social justice' (p19) and argues that the new system will remove 'perverse incentives, balance rights and responsibilities and combine back-to-work help for those who can work with support for those who can't, while respecting rights of disabled people.' (p19) However, the Government is sending out mixed messages:

- On the one hand, it reports that many people who move onto incapacity benefits 'will never return to the workplace, with a devastating impact on themselves [and], their family.' (p32)
- On the other hand, it implies that the generosity of the benefit system prevents people from working 'by offering more money the longer someone is on benefits...' (p24)

Despite the Government's concerns about the generosity of benefits acting as a deterrent to work, high levels of poverty among disabled people indicate that they do not provide an adequate financial safety net. It is hardly surprising that IB (currently a meagre £78.50 a week) is failing to safeguard disabled people from living in poverty. Although it is an 'earnings replacement' benefit, rates are between 16 per cent and 30 per cent of average earnings.[41] While the long-term rate of IB is more generous than JSA, this is an indication of the inadequacies of JSA, not the generosity of IB.[42] As discussed in Chapter 2, 57 per cent of children in workless couple households with at least one disabled parent, many of whom are in receipt of incapacity benefits, are in poverty. The fact that disabled parents are often on these benefits for long periods may result in children experiencing longer, and in some case much longer, spells of being poor.[43]

If moving onto incapacity benefits has 'a devastating impact' on sick or disabled people's lives, then clearly the benefit system does not currently provide security for those who cannot work.

The continuing downward trend in benefits and support for those of working age and outside the labour market is a part of the overall problem. As Barnes and Baldwin argue:

> If the 1980s saw a trend towards increased coverage in benefits for disabled people, this has been balanced by new restrictions and a steady erosion of their living standards... Benefit reforms have reduced the levels of income-replacement benefits, while also tightening eligibility criteria, with damaging effects on independence and autonomy as well as living standards. Disabled people were also badly affected by the 'simplification' of income support after 1988.[44]

There are concerns that the proposed reform is part of a continuing policy to 'tighten' and 'target' disability benefits designed to replace earnings,[45] which has been an integral part of New Labour's approach to social security since 1997, and this may have a negative impact on poverty levels.

Although the Green Paper has indicated that claimants who are on the support component of ESA will receive more money than they do under the current system, there will clearly also be losers. If the incomes of people who are sick or disabled are to be protected and the intractable link between poverty and disability broken, the levels of IB need to be increased significantly for all claimants.

Take-up

The Government argues that IB is just one part of a financial package of support for disabled people (which includes DLA and disability premiums within income support (IS), tax credits and housing benefit). Although additional support for disabled people is triggered by an award of DLA, the DWP acknowledges that 'increasing levels of benefits will not help people unless the benefits are claimed.'[46] However, problems with take-up, particularly among 'hard-to-reach' groups, are an ongoing source of concern.

Although the Green Paper focuses on getting people off benefits and into employment, if child poverty is to be further reduced it is essential that disabled parents (particularly lone parents) and parents with disabled children receive their full benefit entitlement. And yet the 2004 Family and Children Study reports that some lone parents, particularly those with mental health problems on IS, did not realise that they might be eligible for incapacity benefits and so did not claim them. This group (which is disproportionately reliant on benefits and likely to experience severe barriers to employment) must have access to financial security via the benefit system. Low take-up is also a problem with other disadvantaged groups.[47]

Maximised take-up of entitlement is not only a citizen's right, it reduces poverty and may improve health. However, although research indicates that the provision of welfare benefits advice in primary care settings leads to an improvement in health[48] and the Green Paper reports that 'members of the medical profession, and GPs in particular, are often seen as 'gatekeepers' to sick pay and benefits' (p33), CPAG does not believe the importance of independent benefit advice is sufficiently emphasised. An opportunity to improve take-up by linking welfare advice and the medical services has been lost. Furthermore, the need for independent benefits advice will be significantly increased with the introduction of a more complex system, as outlined in the Green Paper. Funding must be made available to ensure that informed and independent advice can be provided.

A more joined-up approach to the provision of benefits advice is needed to support improved take-up. Ensuring that people are in receipt of all the benefits to which they are entitled is essential to safeguard parental health and to keep children out of poverty.

Myths and stigma

Those in receipt of incapacity benefits often feel stigmatised because they are not in paid work, and this is fuelled by myths about the extent of fraudulent claims. CPAG is concerned about some of the language used in the run-up to welfare reform, which risks perpetuating stigma and having a negative impact on take-up. Chapter 4 illustrates that encouraging the public to be vigilant about fraud can have a devastating effect on disabled people's lives.

The Green Paper highlights the low rate of actual fraud and error reporting:

> It is estimated that around 1.2 per cent of expenditure on incapacity benefits is overpaid through fraud and error – this is one of the lowest rates for the benefits system. (p48)

Despite this, the tendency to conflate error and fraud is compounded when the Green Paper sets out detailed information only about how it will deal with fraud. Furthermore, the emphasis on fraud prevention risks exacerbating the fear that disabled people may have of claiming incapacity benefits and being viewed as fraudulent.

As discussed below, we are concerned that the new system will generate higher levels of administrative error, and this may create the erroneous impression of a rise in benefit fraud.

Administration

The administration of incapacity benefits is expensive for the Government, causes significant stress for claimants and CPAG's experience is that errors are common in the administrative process. The overall inadequacy of the administrative system exacerbates the difficulties faced by people who are sick or disabled.

Although the Green Paper asserts that more proactive and frequent engagement with disabled people will 'reduce risk of fraud and error creeping in...' (p48), there are serious concerns about whether the new system will resolve or exacerbate underlying administrative problems given that, although the DWP will provide the 'initial' investment to set up services and Jobcentre Plus will 'administer' the system, the Government intends to 'use private and voluntary sector expertise to provide personal advice and support for individuals to help them back to work.' (p42) We are particularly concerned about the capacity of the voluntary sector and private sector to deliver welfare reform effectively across the country and question whether it is appropriate to involve non-state agencies in decisions about entitlement or to impose benefit conditionality and sanctions on a vulnerable client group.

Furthermore, requiring claimants to attend a series of work-focused interviews and undertake annual personal capability assessments will impose a significant increase in the workload of Jobcentre Plus and other service providers administering the system. This seems illogical at a time of staff cuts within Jobcentre Plus and budgetary restrictions within the DWP. We are not persuaded that the resources allocated will be sufficient to implement a complex new system. We also emphasise the high level of training necessary to deliver an effective and non-stigmatising service to a vulnerable client group.

Poor administrative processes within the benefit system also act as a barrier to employment. We are concerned that the linking rules may not be implemented correctly, particularly when different components of support are administered by different departments, including the DWP, HM Revenue and Customs and local authorities.

Compulsion and sanctions

The Green Paper reports that 'as support is increased, so will the level of conditionality for claimants' (p6) and stipulates that the new benefit 'will be paid to most people in return for undertaking work-related interviews, agreeing an action plan and, as resources allow, participating in some form of work-related activity.' (p4)

We do not believe that the Government has made a compelling case for increased compulsion and/or benefit penalties, and have a number of concerns about a tendency that may plunge the most disadvantaged groups further into poverty. Increased conditionality is neither just, since it risks disadvantaging the most vulnerable children and families, nor is it necessary if the Government believes that 'one million disabled people are willing and able to work'. The Green Paper states that:

> ...if individuals do not participate, as in Pathways to Work, their benefit will be reduced in a series of slices. Ultimately if people continue not to comply, the benefit will return to the level seen during the assessment period. (p44)

Given high levels of poverty among disabled people, we are extremely concerned by the proposed benefit sanctions. We are worried that particularly vulnerable groups of people may be wrongly designated as ready to engage in work-focused activities. If they are not able to do so they will then incur benefit sanctions which will plunge them – and their children if they are parents – further into poverty.

Although the Government argues that it will 'base our reforms on the best possible evidence [and will] build up increased conditionality on the basis of what evidence tells us is most effective...' (p50), international evidence on welfare-to-work programmes for lone parents indicates that in the US, the parents most likely to be sanctioned may be the most vulnerable. Millar and Evans' research on the role of benefit sanctions and time limits in the US established that:

> Compared with other welfare recipients, sanctioned individuals have lower levels of education, less work experience, a high prevalence of health-related barriers to employment, and are more likely to experience several barriers at once.

[They are likely to have] lower household income, are more likely to return to welfare, less likely to be employed and are more likely than non-sanctioned recipients to have personal characteristics, human capital deficits, transportation barriers or personal and family challenges that make them harder to employ.[49]

Evidence from the US on the impact of benefit sanctions on parents with children is a very serious source of concern. One study found that children in families who had been sanctioned, as against those in receipt of social security payments who had not, experienced a one-third higher incidence of past hospitalisations, two-thirds greater risk of 'food insecurity' (for instance, being underweight) and a 90 per cent higher risk of being admitted to hospital on an accident and emergency basis.[50]

Furthermore, the need for compulsion was not indicated by the Pathways to Work pilots. Around 8 per cent of participants on Pathways to Work were volunteers from existing claimants, and accounted for one in five of the people who moved into work.[51] It is worrying that that the Government seems intent on increasing conditionality and introducing sanctions for disabled people without a robust evidence base for its efficacy.

Compulsion also carries an attendant stigma with employers. Using sanctions to force people into work, irrespective of their readiness or ability to do so, is likely to have a negative impact on their health, and could inflame discrimination and exacerbate the underlying reluctance among employers to employ them. Employers are likely to treat people who are encouraged to access work in a mechanistic way as part of employment programmes quite differently from those who actively seek it out.

Benefit sanctions have a negative impact on health outcomes for children, are directly at odds with the Government's desire to implement preventative strategies and have the most negative impact on the poorest people. If the Government simply removed the element of sanction and penalties, and all disabled people were given the opportunity to engage in the new programme of support and rehabilitation, it would obviate the need either to impose sanctions or exclude current claimants. This would reduce the risk of poverty.

Support services

The Pathways pilots and the Green Paper recognise the importance of appropriate services to help disabled people access paid employment –

which is very welcome – but the Green Paper does not refer to the importance of including parental responsibilities when assessing a disabled person's ability to engage in work-focused activities, and/or seek employment.

This is perplexing given that a number of government documents and policy initiatives outline the way in which parenting and additional caring responsibilities impact upon disabled people's care needs and ability to work. For example, *Improving the Life Chances of Disabled People* emphasises that 'recognising the particular needs and circumstances of disabled parents will be vital to the achievement of policy objectives of increasing employment rates and tackling child poverty.'[52]

We recommend that the assessment process and job-search activities take account of the availability of work, transport, childcare, care needs, and educational opportunities. The link between employment opportunities and the availability of childcare, transport, and suitable jobs must be monitored by the DWP.

Rights and responsibilities

Much is made in the Green Paper about rights and responsibilities, and many government initiatives emphasise the importance of choice. However, we are concerned that the increase in responsibilities for some of the most vulnerable groups saps both their choice and their rights. Furthermore, there is nothing to ensure that the imposition of conditions and sanctions will be enforced on all sides. Claimants will be expected to go through all the steps but nothing is being done to ensure, for example, that government agencies honour their responsibilities towards benefit recipients (for example, by ensuring that all personal capability assessments are conducted within 12 weeks), that employers take on a larger number of workers who have been on ESA, or that health trusts provide counselling or other mental health support services.

The Green Paper: the new system in detail

A dual process

As discussed in the Introduction, we have concerns that introducing a new disability benefit with employment and support components (ESA) risks dividing disabled people into 'deserving' and 'undeserving' claimants. Introducing ESA for new claimants while retaining IB for existing claimants means that there will be a three-tiered system in operation (four, including the holding period). Given problems administering the current system, we are concerned that implementing a complex new system may result in an increase in poverty.

Having a dual benefit adds a degree of complexity to the assessment process at the very time that the DWP is investigating benefit simplification. Furthermore, although we accept that the name 'incapacity benefit' sends out a negative message to disabled people and we welcome the emphasis on disabled people's capabilities, given the suspicion with which disability benefit claimants are often viewed, we fear that claimants who receive the employment component who are unable to work or to find a suitable job may find themselves the on the receiving end of even more scrutiny.

Although we accept that disabled people face additional costs, we believe that, if it were effectively administered and reflected additional costs, DLA would provide an appropriate way in which to target additional financial support.

The assessment process

The Government intends to:

> . . . transform the current assessment process . . . so that it provides a professional assessment of an individual's eligibility for financial support, identifies those people who are capable of taking part in work-related activity, identifies people who are so limited by their illness or disability that it would be unreasonable to require them to undertake any form of work-related activity in the foreseeable future. (p38)

The Green Paper specifies that, in the first instance, no judgements will be made about 'the most appropriate benefit for that individual'. However, all claimants will be asked to undertake a work-focused interview after eight weeks (as is the case at present) so that the Government:

> . . . can offer individuals the opportunity to access all the help that is available through Jobcentre Plus, for example, existing employment programmes. In this way, we can ensure that the support is available before benefit assessment is finally determined. (p42)

We welcome the fact that people will be provided with a detailed overview of the sort of support that will be available during the assessment process, and believe that this negates the need for compulsion.

It is not clear how the assessment process will differentiate between people who, with the right support, may be able to work in the future and those who can work now.

Research recently published by the DWP highlights the problems of dividing disabled people into two groups. The author, Richard Berthoud, reports that:

> In practice there are bound to be some people whose employment prospects are not affected by their impairments, and others with virtually no chance of getting a job… If there were a clear polarity between opposite ends of the spectrum, that would… offer an opportunity to identify individuals who were incapable of work. But if most disabled people turned out to be in the middle of the spectrum… the aim of distinguishing between individuals according to whether they were 'capable' or 'incapable' would become both difficult and pointless.[53]

Furthermore, people may want to work, but be unable to do so because of lack of support services generally or because going out to work generates additional care needs at home (if they have caring responsibilities) along with additional childcare needs during the day and in the evening when they may need to recover their energy. People may be deemed to be capable of work, but not be able to get a job because of the lack of, often expensive, specialist equipment in the workplace – for example, for people with sensory impairments. The availability of support, both at home and in the workplace, should be part of an assessment process that gauges an individual's ability to undertake employment.

The personal capability assessment

The Green Paper accepts that the personal capability assessment is 'one of the toughest in the world' and is concerned that it focuses on incapacity rather than capability. (p38) We welcome the focus on a disabled person's capacity rather than her/his incapacity, but we would emphasise that many disabled people view themselves as very capable – as parents, carers and volunteers – yet they may not be able to undertake paid employment. Equating the ability to do paid work with capability risks devaluing people who are unable to work, but who contribute to society in many other ways.

The personal capability assessment is viewed as a negative, sometimes painful, process by disabled people. Given the high number of successful appeals, it is also seen as an ineffective and seemingly arbitrary way of assessing an individual's capability for work, partly because decision makers are often reliant on poor medical assessments. However, although the personal capability assessment certainly needs to be improved, we are concerned that it will take longer if the examining practitioner is to look at both what the claimant can and cannot do, and this has budgetary implications. The DWP will need to ensure that examinations are given adequate time to ensure a proper assessment.

Medical assessments

Eligibility for both components of the new benefit will be determined 'on the basis of evidence provided by medical practitioners...[and] could be assessed by other health professionals as well.' (p39) The medical assessment will not be based on the 'nature of the specific illness or disability the individual has, but on the severity of the impact of that condition on the individual's ability to function.' This is a subtle and fundamentally subjective decision. New medical procedures and additional training will be necessary to support practitioners to make appropriate, informed and much more complex assessments.

We are concerned that the Government's intention 'to reward primary care staff who take active steps to support individuals to remain in or return to work' (p34) may have a negative impact on the attitude of medical practitioners towards people claiming disability benefits, on the attitude of claimants to medical practitioners on whom they rely for support, and on the quality of the supporting medical evidence provided for claimants. Currently, medical evidence can be extremely flimsy and results in many people being wrongly turned down for DLA and IB. We are not convinced that the new system will resolve these problems.

Using GPs both as 'gatekeepers' to benefits and rewarding health professionals who persuade sick or disabled people to access employment may constitute a conflict of interest, and could deter people from seeking medical support or claiming benefits. It may have a negative impact on doctors' attitude to benefit claimants, and may further reduce the quality of medical evidence.

Decision makers

The very poor standard of decision making does not bode well for the new system. Statistics show that IB appeals account for the second highest number of appeals (after DLA) and there is a very high success rate: nearly 75 per cent of IB appeals are found in favour of claimants where they have a representative.[54]

Given significant problems with the current, and relatively more straightforward, decision making process, which simply has to assess the severity of a disabled person's condition, we question whether decision makers will have the expertise, sensitivity and skills to stream as 'capable' or 'incapable' of work a wide spectrum of disabled people with a huge variety of impairments and conditions which have a different impact on them. Much better training will be needed to enable decision makers to decide entitlement. Failure to improve the quality of decision making may generate a higher level of appeals under the new system, which are costly for the state and individuals alike, and may leave vulnerable groups of people without the additional financial support they need.

Inappropriate or incorrect decision making will become even more punitive under the new system because someone who is wrongly placed on the employment component when they should be on the support component could face benefit sanctions. This will increase the risk of poverty and could exacerbate health problems.

Although the Green Paper accepts the need for 'a system that can be flexible to the claimant's changing conditions' (p44), we are concerned that people with fluctuating conditions or mental health problems will find the requirements of the new system onerous. Although personal advisers in Jobcentre Plus have a good reputation, the resources and time allocated to training is unlikely to generate specialist advisers with expertise and understanding of, for example, fluctuating conditions, mental health problems or learning disabilities, and/or the way in which these impact on an individual's ability to work. **Disabled people themselves are best placed to assess whether or not they are capable of work, and their views and opinions should be taken into consideration.**

The basic allowance

We are particularly concerned about placing sick or disabled people on a basic allowance set at JSA rates while their claims are assessed. Four out of every five children in a family receiving JSA are currently left in poverty by a benefit that is supposed to provide a financial 'safety' net.[55] If JSA does not protect non-disabled claimants from poverty, the impact on sick or disabled claimants (who incur significant additional costs) is likely to be much worse. The relationship between ill-health and poverty indicates that a dramatic reduction in income at the time of onset of disability or ill-health will exacerbate underlying health problems and may undermine rehabilitation attempts during the early months.[56] Placing sick or disabled people on JSA rates will force a particularly vulnerable group of people into poverty. This is likely to have an adverse impact on their health and undermine their ability to engage in work-focused activities or access paid employment.

The Green Paper suggests that young disabled people will receive an even lower level of the basic allowance, as young people currently do on JSA. Even if they are awarded the employment or support component, their overall income will be less than disabled adults because they are starting from a lower basic level of support. This is neither just nor likely to prove effective at getting young people into work. It will place a marginalised group, many of whom have little education or training and face major barriers to employment, at an additional disadvantage at a point at which, as the Green Paper stipulates, the Government should be 'helping a smooth transition into adulthood.' (p49)

The Prime Minister recently commented that the low number of children in care receiving decent GCSE results 'was appalling'.[57] We fear that this aspect of the Green Paper is likely to have a particularly negative impact on care leavers who are disproportionately likely to be disabled.[58] Placing disabled young people who face significant barriers to employment at a financial disadvantage is a profoundly disturbing aspect of the Green Paper which runs counter to government policies on prevention, child poverty and support for families.

The employment component

Claimants who are awarded the employment component of the new allowance will be expected to draw up an action plan, which will include activities such as work tasters, managing health in work, improving employability, jobsearch assistance, and stabilising life. We welcome the fact that voluntary work will be possible. However, although 'childcare options' are included in the list, there is little recognition of disabled people's parenting or caring responsibilities. This is worrying, given that the Government has on other occasions emphasised that parental responsibilities must be taken into consideration when assessing a disabled adult's care needs.[59]

We are concerned about the length of time an individual will be expected to engage in work-focused activities if paid employment is not forthcoming. An evaluation of the Pathways to Work pilots indicates that some participants felt disappointed and frustrated at the lack of support and the difficulties they experienced finding appropriate jobs, perhaps because their expectations were unrealistic, or because their health had deteriorated.[60] We fear that the new system may arouse false expectations about employment opportunities, which may lead to disappointment and disengagement. Engaging in perpetual work-focused activities which do not result in employment is likely to be demoralising and possibly have a negative impact on people's health.

The support component

The Green Paper argues that 'for people with the most severe functional limitations, it would be unreasonable to expect that they engage in work-related activity.' (p39) They will be placed on the support component of ESA and will not be expected to engage in work-focused activities or to seek employment, although they may choose to do so. We welcome the element of choice within the support component and the commitment that people will receive a higher rate of financial support, but we believe that this should apply to all disabled claimants.

Existing claimants

The Green Paper states that:

> The benefit structure and conditionality requirements...will only apply to new claimants. Existing claimants will remain on their current benefit level... [However,] existing claimants will have more manageable conditions, which may have changed or improved while they have been on benefits...[and the Government proposes] to work more proactively with this group. (p47)

We have a number of concerns about existing claimants. On the one hand, if the rates of ESA are higher than IB, existing claimants, who may be long-term recipients of benefit and may have more intractable health conditions, could be financially worse off than new claimants. On the other hand, given that there will be winners and losers under the new system, some disabled people with more severe conditions may end up worse off than existing claimants. This is an inequitable situation. It is important that disabled people receive the financial support they need to cover additional needs – irrespective of whether they are new or existing claimants – and that no one is actively disadvantaged by a system that is supposed to provide greater financial security.

Delivery

Effective delivery is fundamental to the success of the Green Paper, which emphasises that implementing a radical programme of reform requires more than just legislative and policy change but a delivery network that is effective, accessible and flexible.' (p74) The Green Paper argues that:

> In taking forward our reforms we need to ensure that we provide the best possible service for our clients, the best possible recruits for employers, and the best possible value for the taxpayer. (p75)

The proposals are ambitious and will be challenging to deliver. CPAG has yet to be convinced that the Government is in a position to administrate the proposed reforms effectively or efficiently. Failure to deliver will neither increase the employment rate nor reduce child poverty.
 We also have serious reservations about the Government's desire to 'draw on the wealth of experience of those working in other sectors' and will

be 'looking for greater involvement on the part of voluntary sector and private providers in the future reform agenda.' (p75) Although it makes sense to draw on the experience and expertise of both sectors, CPAG has a number of key concerns about this proposal, including the risk of a postcode lottery, the loss of innovation and independence within the voluntary sector, problems with accountability and issues around inspection and monitoring.

Resources

An ambitious welfare reform programme is being planned at a time of considerable disquiet over the proposed staff cuts in Jobcentre Plus and the Budget announcement of year-on-year cuts of 5 per cent in the DWP.

An additional £360 million has been announced to fund the Green Paper proposals to roll out Pathways to Work. It is not clear where these resources will come from beyond that this is to be funded from existing DWP budgets – and the £360 million does not appear to include either setting up costs for providers or return-to-work credit. It is equally not clear if the costs of delivering Pathways to Work will increase as those further from the labour market begin to access it.

Long-term benefits reform

The Government argues that 'the reforms set out in the Green Paper will reduce much of the complexity surrounding existing benefits for those facing health problems and disability'. Given the complexities illustrated above, we are at a loss to see how this can possibly be the case.

CPAG does not reject the more radical approaches to benefit reform suggested in the Green Paper, including the single working-age benefit, but we are concerned about the effective implementation of such a scheme, particularly if it continues to be based on means-testing. More importantly, improvements should be implemented within the DWP and other departments to improve the management and administration of the current system. The proposed reform of IB adds an additional layer of complexity which is at odds with plans to simplify the system and which may be all the more challenging to deliver effectively.

Complexity brings a number of problems which leave vulnerable groups without the benefits to which they are entitled and renders them susceptible to poverty. But it is surely more important to address issues such as low take-up, increased administrative and claimant error, over-

and underpayments, poor and inconsistent decision making, and delays, than to introduce a complex new system that may make the situation worse.[61]

Conclusion

Welfare reform needs to be viewed within wider government policy initiatives. The welcome implementation of the 1995 Disability Discrimination Act and publication of *Improving the Life Chances of Disabled People* illustrate the Government's recognition of the fact that addressing the needs of disabled people is the responsibility of a wide range of government departments and other agencies, and this perspective has been consolidated by the new cross-government Office for Disability Issues.

However, the Green Paper is trying to do many things. An ambitious approach which outlines significant changes to the treatment of various groups and areas of policy has resulted in a document in which the direction is somewhat confused and not always consistent. There are areas – for instance around the importance of supporting parenting – where the welfare reform agenda does not join up with other agendas in government. CPAG is concerned that the Green Paper does not reflect an interdepartmental perspective, and sometimes ignores policies emanating from other departments.

Disabled people face significant barriers to work, and initiatives that resolve structural barriers (such as insufficient childcare, low skills, poorly paid jobs and disadvantaged neighbourhoods), address discrimination and put support services in place to assist more disabled people access paid employment are essential prerequisites for success. However, CPAG fears that welfare reform does not necessarily complement and may actually undermine policies designed to tackle such issues. We believe that it would be more effective to address benefit inadequacy (both to tackle poverty and to prevent ill-health), offer supportive routes into work (such as by extending the Pathways to Work scheme) and to overcome barriers to work and employer discrimination, rather than to introduce a complex new system that will be expensive to administer and may leave some disabled people worse off.

Perhaps more fundamentally, we are not persuaded that IB is the problem that rhetoric implies. Although the number of people applying for IB has increased, in part because of an increase in the number of women accessing paid employment and an ageing population, the number of people receiving IB has in fact been falling. Between 1995 and 2005, the total number of beneficiaries of IB fell from 2.2 million to 1.7 million. The DWP annual report, *Opportunity for All* states:

> The volume of people making a new claim for incapacity benefit has fallen by over a quarter since 1997; and after more than two decades of substantial growth the working-age incapacity benefit caseload has fallen slightly to 2.74 million, a fall of around 41,000 over the year to May 2005.[62]

If the overall trend is going in the right direction, it is hard to know why the Government feels the need to change the structure of the entire system. Such an ambitious programme of reform is particularly perplexing given the Government's aspiration to simplify the benefit system, to reduce the workload – and costs – within the DWP, and to ensure that disabled people receive the financial support they need to safeguard themselves and their children from poverty.

Notes

1 CPAG's submission can be downloaded from www.cpag.org.uk

2 Department for Work and Pensions, *A New Deal for Welfare: empowering people to work*, The Stationery Office, p29, para 19

3 The *Every Child Matters* Green Paper was published in September 2003, and the public consultation ran until December 2003. *Every Child Matters: change for children* was delivered by ministers responsible for services for children and young people at the Department for Education and Skills, Department of Health, Department for Work and Pensions, HM Treasury, Office of the Deputy Prime Minister, Department for Environment, Food and Rural Affairs, Department of Trade and Industry, Ministry of Defence, Department for Constitutional Affairs, Home Office, Department for Culture, Media and Sport. *Every Child Matters* is available from www.dfes.gov.uk/everychildmatters. The consultation and supporting documents are available from www.everychildmatters.gov.uk/key-documents/

4 HM Treasury, *Child Poverty Review*, The Stationery Office, 2004

5 Cabinet Office, Prime Minister's Strategy Unit, *Improving the Life Chances of Disabled People*, 2005 (a joint report with the Department for Work and Pensions, Department of Health, Department for Education and Skills and Office of the Deputy Prime Minister)

6 G Palmer, J Carr and P Kenway, *Monitoring Poverty and Social Exclusion*, Joseph Rowntree Foundation and New Policy Institute, 2005

7 See J Carvel, 'Wealth Brings 17 More Years of Health' in the *Guardian*, 25 February 2005. Discussing findings from a recent report from the Office for National Statistics, the *Guardian* reports that a poorer man's healthy life expectancy was only 49.4 years, nearly 17 years less than a man from a prosperous ward. A woman's healthy life expectancy is 51.7 in deprived wards and 68.5 years in the most prosperous wards.

8 H Stickland and R Olsen, 'Children with Disabled Parents' in G Preston (ed), *At Greatest Risk: the children most likely to be poor*, CPAG, 2005

9 See T Burchardt, *Being and Becoming: social exclusion and the onset of disability*, CASEreport 21, Centre for Analysis of Social Exclusion, 2003

10 See note 5, p25

11 S Jenkins and J Rigg, *Disability and Disadvantage: selection, onset and duration effects*, CASEpaper74, Centre for Analysis of Social Exclusion, 2003, p11

12 See note 6

13 See note 5

14 See note 6

15 See note 6, pp14-15

16 TUC, *Sicknote Britain? Countering an urban legend*, TUC Economic and Social Affairs, 2005

17 See note 8

18 One Parent Families, *Meeting the Target: how can the Government achieve a 70 per cent employment rate for lone parents?*, One Parent Families, 2005

19 Department for Work and Pensions, *Households Below Average Income 1994/95–2004/05*, Corporate Document Services, 2006, Table 4.7

20 See note 8, p138

21 N Lyon, M Barnes and D Sweiry, *Families with Children in Britain: findings from the 2004 Families and Children Study* (FACS), Corporate Document Services, 2006

22 One Parent Families, *One Parent Families Today: the facts*, One Parent Families, 2005

23 See, for example, J Casebourne and L Britton, *Lone Parents, Health and Work*, DWP Research Report 214, 2004

24 See note 19, Table 4.7

25 See note 4

26 Further information about CPAG's specific concerns about the impact of the new system on benefits can be downloaded from www.cpag.org.uk

27 L Elliott, 'Unemployment Heads for 1m by Summer' in the *Guardian*, 13 April 2006. Citing recent statistics issued by the Office for National Statistics, the *Guardian* reports a jump of 12,600 in unemployment in March.

28 B Blythe, *Incapacity Benefit Reforms: Pathways to Work Pilots' performance and analysis*, DWP Working Paper 26, 2006 states 'Incapacity Benefit Leavers: around an eight percentage point increase in the IB six month off-flow rates in the Pilot districts.'(p8)

29 C Mackay and others, 'Management Standards and Work-related Stress in the UK: policy background and science' in *Work and Stress*, Vol 18, No.2, 2004, pp91-112

30 Department of Health White Paper, *Choosing Health: making healthy choices easier*, 2004, p159

31 See note 30, p159

32 See note 19, Table 4.4

33 Social Exclusion Unit, *Mental Health and Social Exclusion*, Office of the Deputy Prime Minister 2004, p3

34 See note 33, p3

35 See K Higginbottom, 'Down but not Out' in the *Guardian*, 15 April 2006

36 T Burchardt, *The Education and Employment of Disabled Young People: frustrated ambition*, Joseph Rowntree Foundation, 2005

37 See G Cooke, *Realising the Childcare Revolution*, 4Children, 2004

38 Department for Work and Pensions, *Opportunity for All: seventh annual report*, The Stationery Office, 2005, p124

39 R Chote, C Emmerson, D Miles and Z Oldfield, *The IFS Green Budget: January 2005*, Institute for Fiscal Studies, 2005 reports that 'the majority of recipients are families on middle or average incomes, with around 7 per cent of families in each of the third to seventh deciles receiving the childcare tax credit... The beneficiaries from both the programme as a whole and the changes announced in the *Pre-Budget Report* are mostly in the middle of the income distribution... our data suggest that some of the richest 10 per cent of families are benefiting from the childcare tax credit... This means that the childcare tax credit has almost no direct impact on child poverty as measured by the Government.' (p154)

40 Letter to CPAG from Disability and Carers Service, Department for Work and Pensions, 21 April 2006

41 For further information see T Burchardt, *The Evolution of Disability Benefits in the UK: re-weighting the basket*, CASEpaper 26, Centre for Analysis of Social Exclusion, 1999 and note 9

42 Department for Work and Pensions, *Households Below Average Income 1994/05-2003/04*, Corporate Document Services, 2005 indicates the woeful inadequacies of both IS and JSA. According to the DWP, 'Those families living in households in receipt of jobseeker's allowance (JSA) were heavily skewed towards the bottom of the distribution, with around three-quarters in the bottom quintile. Children living in families claiming housing benefit (HB) and/or income

support were predominantly in the bottom two quintiles.' HBAI reveals that the risk of children in a household in receipt of JSA living below 60 per cent of median income is 64 per cent (BHC) and 73 per cent (AHC). (pp37 and 51)

43 See note 8

44 See, for example, H Barnes and S Baldwin 'Social Security, Poverty and Disability' in J Ditch (ed), *Introduction to Social Security*, Routledge, 1999, pp156-176

45 See note 41

46 Department for Work and Pensions, *Opportunity for All: fifth annual report*, The Stationery Office, 2003

47 See K Roberts and D Lawton, *Reaching its Target? Disability living allowance for children*, Social Policy Report 9, Social Policy Research Unit, University of York, 1999 and R Chamba, W Adham, M Hirst, MD Dawton and B Beresford, *On the Edge: minority ethnic families caring for a severely disabled child*, The Policy Press, 1999

48 See, for example, S Abbott and L Hobby, *What is the Impact on Individual Health of Services in Primary Health Care Settings which Offer Welfare Benefit Advice?*, Health and Community Care Research Unit, 2003

49 See J Millar and M Evans (eds), *Lone Parents and Employment: international comparisons of what works*, Centre for the Analysis of Social Policy, 2003, p51

50 See, for example, A Skalicky and J T Cook, *The Impact of Welfare Sanctions on the Health of Infants and Toddlers*, The Children's Sentinel Nutrition Assessment Program, 2002

51 See note 34. 'There were a total of 147,950 starts to the Pathways to Work process… 11,200 are currently identifiable as voluntary participants' (7.6 per cent). 'There were a total of 19,550 Pathways job entries to end of August… 3,010 were from the voluntary customer group' (15.5 per cent). 'This means that jobs from voluntary customers are making a significant contribution to Pathways performance.' (pp11 and 16)

52 See note 5, p83

53 R Berthoud, *The Employment Rates of Disabled People*, DWP Research Report 298, 2006

54 Department for Work and Pensions, *Quarterly Appeal Tribunal Statistics*, June 2005

55 See note 42

56 R Berthoud, *The Profile of Exits from Incapacity-related Benefits over Time*, DWP Working Paper 17, 2004

57 See P Wintour, 'Blair Admits Failing Most Needy Children' in the *Guardian*, 16 May 2006

58 See Office for National Statistics, *The Mental Health of Young People Looked After by Local Authorities in England*, Office for National Statistics, 2003. This research indicated that 'among young people aged between 5 and 17 years who were looked after by local authorities in England, 45 per cent were assessed as having a mental disorder.' (With similar rates in Scotland (45 per cent) and Wales (49 per cent)). Among 11 to 15-year-olds, about 68 per cent were assessed as having a mental disorder. Two-thirds of all looked-after children were reported by their carers to have at least one physical complaint.' 'Over three-quarters of children with a mental disorder had at least one physical complaint compared with just over half of the children who were assessed as not having a mental disorder.'

59 Department of Health, *Fair Access to Care Services: guidance on eligibility criteria for adult social care*, 2005 stresses that 'in the course of assessing an individual's needs, councils should recognise that adults, who have parenting responsibilities for a child under 18 years, may require help with these responsibilities.' (p2)

60 A Corden, K Nice and R Sainsbury, *Incapacity Benefit Reforms Pilot: findings from a longitudinal panel of clients*, DWP Research Report 259, 2005

61 Further information about CPAG's views on the simplification of the system is outlined in our response to the Public Accounts Committee, which can be downloaded from www.cpag.org.uk.

62 See note 38, p51

Conclusion
Gabrielle Preston

The Government is committed to reducing child poverty, and has placed support for parents and carers at the heart of its approach to improving outcomes for children. The need for better universal and targeted services for families and children has also been placed at the forefront of policy – for example, in *Every Child Matters*.[1] The most critical judgement of policy success is its impact on children, and yet their needs have not been specifically addressed in the Green Paper. While the needs of disabled parents are considered in government analyses of child poverty (for example, the *Child Poverty Review*)[2] and the child poverty agenda is an integral part of the Government's desire to increase employment among disabled people (see, for example, the Department for Work and Pensions' annual poverty report, *Opportunity for All*)[3], the Green Paper on welfare reform does not consider the potential impact of benefit sanctions and conditionality – or the risk of moving disabled parents into low-paid employment – on child poverty. Furthermore, the recently published *Support for Parents: the best start for children* does not consider the needs of disabled parents.[4] If 'joined-up services' are to be a reality, welfare reform must place the needs of children with disabled parents at the forefront of legislative requirements. Inadequate benefit income and in-work poverty – both of which generate child poverty – must be given a higher prominence in the debate on incapacity benefits, as must the reality of service provision.

Routes out of poverty?

Employment

This publication raises a number of issues about the efficacy of focusing on employment as the primary route out of poverty for everyone and clearly reveals that disabled people continue to be disadvantaged in the labour market. We are concerned that the new proposals outlined in the Green

Paper will pressurise the most vulnerable disabled people, who may have low educational qualifications and poor health, into low-paid, unrewarding and stressful jobs, which may exacerbate their condition and may not leave them better off financially. This is at odds with the Government's commitment to eradicate poverty. The Government's message about greater flexibility in employment structures and working conditions must become a reality if it is to offer genuine opportunities to disabled people.

There are other reasons why work might not pay for disabled people. In Chapter 4 disabled parents highlight the fact that moving into employment not only generates additional costs for employers, but it increases individuals' care and mobility costs. And yet there is evidence that disability living allowance (DLA), which is designed to meet some of the additional costs incurred by disabled people, is sometimes downrated or removed when a disabled person moves into work. This means that income (often low income) from employment is being sapped by additional costs, while financial support to cover those costs is removed. This situation undermines the efficacy of work as a route out of poverty for disabled people.

More should be done to ensure that employers provide a safe and healthy working environment, which is appropriate and supportive for all disabled people, and which helps prevent the onset of sickness or ill-health. For the moment, however, work routines and structures are often not sufficiently flexible to enable either parents or disabled people – particularly disabled parents – to work. For disabled parents, there is the additional challenge of juggling health needs, parenting needs and the demands of work.

We are concerned that the Government's focus on the merits of paid work, which has dominated policy since 1997, makes people who are not in work feel worthless. Much more emphasis should be placed on the contribution and participation of disabled people, irrespective of their ability to access paid employment. Many disabled people work as volunteers or carers, or run service user groups, and yet are deemed to be out of work because they are not being paid. The Green Paper, with its focus on drawing people into employment, may perpetuate entrenched stereotypes.

Benefits

Benefit adequacy and the importance of ensuring that disabled people receive the benefits to which they are entitled are essential to protect those who are unable to work from living in poverty. And yet these have received scant attention in the Green Paper. Indeed, the Government is sending out very mixed messages on the benefit system. On the one hand, the Green Paper reports that many people who move onto incapacity benefits 'will never return to the workplace, with a devastating impact on themselves [and], their family.' On the other hand, it implies that the generosity of the benefit system prevents people from working 'by offering more money the longer someone is on benefits...' If moving onto incapacity benefits has 'a devastating impact' upon sick or disabled people's lives, then clearly the benefit system is not currently providing security for those who cannot work. We do not believe that the 'generosity' of benefits is a deterrent to employment.

In fact, as David Piachaud points out in *At Greatest Risk: the children most likely to be poor*:

> The 'safety net' provided by the State is still far below its own poverty level. Indeed, the relative levels of the safety net for most families remains lower in 2004/05 than in 1994/95. All that can be said about this fact is that this situation is inconsistent, indefensible and shameful.[5]

CPAG estimates that the current gap between the safety net and the poverty line is 33.8 per cent for a couple with two children aged 5 and 11, and 20.4 per cent for a single person with two children aged 5 and 11.[6]

Low levels of income support sap overall household income and draw the most disadvantaged children into poverty. Given the many barriers that disabled parents and lone parents face to employment, many will continue to be dependent on benefits. Adequate benefits not only protect workless households from poverty, but they provide a route into work. Benefit adequacy must be an integral part of welfare reform.

We are concerned that an already inadequate benefit system may be rendered worse by the implementation of benefit sanctions for disabled people who do not fulfil the work-search requirements. The Government has introduced a number of improvements to disability benefits, which have helped to lift many children out of poverty. The introduction of benefit sanctions could jeopardise the progress that has been made and flies in the face of the Government's child poverty strategy. The implementation of sanctions may have a negative impact upon disabled parents who have young children or who have limited energy as a result of their impairments and who are, therefore, not seeking paid employment, and will disadvantage parents with mental health problems, learning disabilities or fluctuating conditions. Reducing parental income to jobseeker's allowance (JSA) rates will plunge these parents and their children further into poverty.

Young disabled people will also be seriously disadvantaged by the proposed changes. Although much is made in the Green Paper about increasing the expectations of disabled people, the high aspirations in young people with disabilities, as discussed in Chapter 3, are often undermined by low educational attainment and high unemployment. And yet proposals contained in the Green Paper place this group of disabled people at a financial disadvantage because they will be placed on the lower rate of the new employment and support allowance (ESA), set at JSA rates. Even if they are awarded a top-up of the employment or support component, their incomes will be lower than other disabled people. The Government accepts that disabled young people – many of whom are care leavers – are some of the most disadvantaged groups in the UK. This is a profoundly disturbing aspect of the Green Paper, which runs counter to government policies on prevention of cycles of disadvantage, child poverty and support for families.

The Government has also publicly and repeatedly acknowledged that fraud among incapacity benefit (IB) claimants is extremely low. Addressing a Social Market Foundation seminar, Jane Kennedy MP stated:

> While it is taken very seriously where it occurs, fraud in the sense of blatant misrepresentation of condition or claiming whilst working full time appears exceptional for this customer group and the level of measured fraud is extremely low.[7]

And yet, despite an overall positive tone, the Green Paper emphasises that:

> There may be a minority of claimants who, although able to undertake some work, will seek to prolong unnecessarily their time on the protected level of incapacity benefits...[therefore we will introduce] randomly selected, ad hoc case checks to be carried out by a dedicated team which will be specially created for this purpose.

Although such a paragraph may have been inserted to mollify the 'benefit fraudster' brigade, it risks further worrying and alienating sick and disabled people who feel that they are likely to be treated with suspicion. Stigma – and the belief that individuals are not disabled – are major factors that deter people from claiming the incapacity benefits to which they are entitled. By pandering to the public's obsession with fraud, the Government risks inflaming, rather than addressing, misguided and prejudiced beliefs that many claimants of incapacity benefits are frauds.

Service provision

The Government views the provision of appropriate and accessible services as an integral part of its strategy to lift people out of poverty. The Pathways to Work pilots and the Green Paper recognise the importance of putting appropriate services in place to help disabled people access paid employment. However, the provision of adequate support for disabled people is far from effective and is the source of considerable stress. The implementation of *Fairer Charging Policies: for home care and other non-residential services*, designed to reduce inconsistencies and discrepancies in local authority charging systems, highlighted ongoing problems with support services for disabled people.[8] Disabled people have to pay for additional support services. Disabled parents in this book emphasise that, if they access employment, their care needs, as well as their costs, will rise, and this must be recognised within the welfare reform programme.

A recent report published by the Department of Health, *Fair Access to Care Services: guidance on eligibility criteria for adult social care*, stresses that:

> In the course of assessing an individual's needs, councils should recognise that adults, who have parenting responsibilities for a child under 18 years, may require help with these responsibilities.[9]

Improving the Life Chances of Disabled People acknowledges the barriers to employment faced by disabled parents and emphasises that:

> Recognising the particular needs and circumstances of disabled parents will be vital to the achievement of policy objectives of increasing employment rates and tackling child poverty.[10]

However, there is no recognition in the Green Paper about the way in which parenting and additional caring responsibilities impact upon a disabled adult's ability to undertaken paid employment.

Delivery issues

Welfare reform is an extremely costly venture and we are seriously concerned about delivery issues, particularly given proposed staff cuts of 30,000 staff within Jobcentre Plus and the further 5 per cent reduction in the Department for Work and Pensions' (DWP) budget announced in Budget 2006.[11] The Government has allocated £360 million for the roll out of Pathways to Work and the implementation of the Green Paper's proposals on incapacity benefits. We are concerned that £360 million will not be sufficient to maintain the high level of support currently on offer in the Pathways pilots. As it is, the Pathways pilots may have engaged easier to help groups and if all new claimants are involved, costs will be higher. The DWP acknowledges that, to begin with, resources are not sufficient to include existing claimants.

Increasing the number of work-focused interviews and personal capability assessments will be expensive and labour intensive. An increasing reliance on medical practitioners also has resource implications. Although the Green Paper emphasises the importance of working with the health services, the recent budgetary crisis within the NHS does not bode well for improved service provision, or an improvement in the quality of medical assessments.

Is welfare reform necessary?

Given that the number of IB claimants is gradually falling and the incidence of fraud is very low, we question whether a totally new system is necessary. Improving the administration of the current system to ensure that sick and disabled people who are at risk of poverty receive the benefits to which they are entitled, addressing benefit adequacy so that it safeguards parents and children from poverty, and revising and improving the assessment process to ensure that it does not act as a deterrent to work, could all be achieved without introducing a complex, new and expensive system. The Government could roll out the Pathways to Work pilots and encourage more disabled people to access paid employment without legislative change. Furthermore, setting an ambitious and seemingly arbitrary target of getting one million disabled people into work may send out the message that many disabled people are, indeed, currently fraudulent beneficiaries of disability benefits.

Recommendations

- The provision of better quality, better paid jobs is crucial to reduce work-related ill-health. It is not known, however, what sort of jobs disabled people who participated in the Pathways pilots moved into. **The Government must monitor the quality and sustainability of jobs that disabled people are accessing, and ensure that good quality jobs are available to allow disabled people to fulfil their potential and which reflect their skill levels.**
- For those disabled adults who cannot work, state benefits are the only route out of poverty. If tackling child poverty is to be successful and health inequalities reduced, the current inadequacy of benefits for this group must be addressed. We believe that a **significant investment in support – not benefit sanctions – is a prerequisite of success.**
- CPAG is concerned at the failure of the proposed measures on welfare reform to take a holistic approach to disability and to address the particular needs of disabled parents. We fear that the failure to take family responsibilities into consideration may disadvantage a particularly vulnerable group of children, which could undermine the Government's strategy on the eradication of child poverty. **A disabled person's family, caring and parental responsibilities must be taken into consideration when assessing her/his ability to undertake work-focused activities to ensure that these do not have a negative impact on her/his children.**
- The Green Paper does not reflect a number of government recommendations and regulations on assessing the care needs of disabled adults, even though this is an integral part of the strategy to help more disabled people access paid employment. **Joined-up policy that reflects and reinforces policies and recommendations on child poverty issued by a range of government departments must be incorporated within welfare reform. The *Every Child Matters* agenda must be at the forefront.**
- Disabled people feel discriminated against, both because of their disability and because of their reliance on benefits. Although the Green Paper argues that 'we need to change the current culture and raise the expectations of employers, health professionals and disabled people themselves...', **policy initiatives are unlikely to improve employment opportunities for disabled people unless they are accompanied by more positive messages.**

- Disabled children and young people continue to be disadvantaged in the educational system, and disability is not discussed in an open and informed manner in schools and colleges. **Much more work needs to be done to overcome discrimination in society at large, and among employers in particular.**
- The Green Paper proposes that young people aged 16 to 25 will receive a lower rate of the basic allowance of ESA. Even if they are awarded the top-up of the employment or support component, their incomes will be lower than those of other disabled people. The Government accepts that disabled young people – many of whom are care leavers – are some of the most disadvantaged groups in the UK. **Young disabled people incur the same sort of disability-related costs as disabled adults and should receive an equivalent level of financial support.**
- Research on health inequalities indicates that living on a low income significantly increases the risk of disability or ill-health. People who are already out of work and reliant on benefits are more likely to become disabled. Many people who move onto IB are already benefit claimants.[12] **A financial safety net must be provided for disabled people who are unable to work, or who are severely disadvantaged in the labour market. Reviewing benefit adequacy and take-up must be an integral part of welfare reform.**
- People who have become sick or developed a disability need additional financial support to help them and their families adjust. Setting the basic allowance of ESA at JSA levels may compound underlying health problems, and could plunge parents and children into poverty. **The level of financial support within the new system, including the basic allowance and the employment and support components, needs to be sufficient to keep disabled people and their children out of poverty.**
- Research indicates that disadvantaged groups, particularly from Black and minority ethnic communities who also experience high levels of unemployment, are least likely to apply for and/or receive incapacity benefits. **We are concerned that the most vulnerable groups who have the greatest difficulties accessing the current system will be most disadvantaged by a new and more complex system with higher levels of conditionality and penalties.**
- Although DLA is not an integral part of welfare reform, disabled parents report that their mobility and care needs go up when they move into work. Ensuring that disabled people receive the benefits to which they are enti-

tled, and that those benefits cover their additional costs (for the moment DLA does not take parenting tasks and roles into consideration) must be an integral part of welfare reform. **The additional costs of being a disabled person with parenting responsibilities, and the additional costs of employment must be recognised and addressed.**

- Although the Green Paper is designed to be part and parcel of the Government's programme of benefit simplification, **we are concerned that having a dual benefit will add a layer of complexity which will increase the potential for administrative error and may leave disabled people without the support they need.**
- The introduction of sanctions may disadvantage the most vulnerable groups, including people with mental health problems, learning disabilities and fluctuating conditions. **The efficacy of increased conditionality, compulsion and sanctions must be reviewed in the light of their potential impact on child poverty.**
- Inadequate, fragmented services consolidate financial difficulties on a daily basis. We urge the Government to implement the recommendations outlined in *Improving the Life Chances of Disabled People*:

> It will be the collective responsibility of all government departments to ensure that the recommendations in the report are taken forward.[13]

The Government must improve service delivery for all disabled people, irrespective of whether they are in employment or not. Services must take disabled people's parenting responsibilities into consideration.

- Disabled people are the experts on their condition, capabilities and ability to undertake employment. **It is crucial that service users be consulted at every level during the consultative process on welfare reform.**
- CPAG believes that more emphasis should be put on the preventative measures needed to pre-empt the onset of ill-health or disability – both of which are closely linked with poverty and deprivation. **Welfare reform must be an integral part of government initiatives to address the underlying social, educational and financial problems that may increase the risk of disability, exacerbate health inequalities and undermine its ability to redress intergenerational cycles of deprivation.**

Notes

1 *Every Child Matters: change for children*, was delivered by ministers responsible for services for children and young people at the Department for Education and Skills, Department of Health, Department for Work and Pensions, HM Treasury, Office of the Deputy Prime Minister, Department for Environment, Food and Rural Affairs, Department of Trade and Industry, Ministry of Defence, Department for Constitutional Affairs, Home Office and Department for Culture, Media and Sport.

2 HM Treasury, *Child Poverty Review*, The Stationery Office, 2004 reports that 'specialised support for families in very specific circumstances such as disabled parents, parents with mental health problems, or parents suffering from addition will be expanded. This support will ensure that links are made between the services being provided to an adult who is a parent and the needs of their children… Looking ahead the Government will consider how to improve integration between adult and children's social services… This will include considering how best to promulgate the message that parenting roles and responsibilities should be routinely considered as part of the assessment for community care services.' (p63)

3 Department for Work and Pensions, *Opportunity for All: seventh annual report*, The Stationery Office, 2005

4 HM Treasury and Department for Education and Skills, *Support for Parents: the best start for children*, 2005, identifies disabled children and children with special educational needs as two of the four most vulnerable groups of children for whom 'outcomes…have not always improved as much as they need in order to put their life chances on an equal footing with those of their peers.' (p50) Given that a significant number of disabled adults also have disabled children, this is very welcome.

5 D Piachaud, 'Child Poverty: an overview' in G Preston (ed), *At Greatest Risk: the children most likely to be poor*, CPAG, 2005, p17

6 These figures are drawn from an analysis undertaken by CPAG using after housing cost figures from Department for Work and Pensions, *Households Below Average Income 1994/95-2004/05*, Corporate Document Services, 2006

7 J Kennedy, speech at Social Market Foundation seminar,14 December 2004

8 See, for example, P Thompson 'Fair for Whom?' in *Disability Rights Bulletin*, Disability Alliance, Summer 2004, pp2-6, which reports that 'the maximum charges reported range from £23.50 to £400 a week.'

9 Department of Health, *Fair Access to Care Services: guidance on eligibility criteria for adult social care*, 2005

10 Cabinet Office, Prime Minister's Strategy Unit, *Improving the Life Chances of Disabled People*, 2005 (a joint report with the Department for Work and Pensions, Department of Health, Department for Education and Skills and Office of the Deputy Prime Minister), p83

11 HM Treasury, Budget 2006, specifies 'the Department for Work and Pensions, HM Treasury and Customs, HM Treasury and the Cabinet Office have already agreed to deliver ambitious value for money reforms over the CSR period enabling them to continue improving services within Departmental Expenditure Limits (DEL) that will continue to fall by 5 per cent in real terms per year in 2008-09, 2009-10 and 2010-11.' (p136)

12 Department for Work and Pensions, *A New Deal for Welfare: empowering people to work*, The Stationery Office, 2006, confirms that 'a significant proportion of new claimants come onto incapacity benefits from employment.' (p25)

13 See note 10